Head, Heart, and Hands

Head, Heart, and Hands

CELEBRATING THE JOY OF NURSING

Nancy Duphily

Fitchburg State University

cognella

SAN DIEGO

Bassim Hamadeh, CEO and Publisher
Amanda Martin, Executive Publisher
Alverne Ball, Project Editor
Rachel Kahn, Production Editor
Jess Estrella, Senior Graphic Designer
Laura Duncan, Licensing Specialist
Tiffany Mok, Senior Content Marketing Specialist
Natalie Piccotti, Director of Marketing
Kassie Graves, Senior Vice President, Editorial
Alia Bales, Director of Project Editorial & Production

Printed in the United States of America.

This book is dedicated to

students, colleagues, family, and friends

past, present, and future

my greatest teachers

Nancy Hinchcliffe Duphily

March 2026

BRIEF CONTENTS

Acknowledgments xv

Prologue xvii

Part I Introduction 1

Chapter 1 Contemplating a Career in Nursing 3

Part II Critical Incidents 19

Chapter 2 The Critical Incident: Change 21

Chapter 3 Caring 29

Chapter 4 Integrating Theory and Evidence-Based Practice 37

Chapter 5 Communication and Culture 43

Chapter 6 Civility 53

Chapter 7 Lifelong Learning 59

Chapter 8 Resilience 67

Part III Looking Ahead 75

Chapter 9 Growing Our Own 77

Chapter 10 Building a Culture of Safety 91

Chapter 11 Cultural Literacy 103

Chapter 12 Informatics Literacy: Strengthening Informatics and Health Information Literacy 115

Chapter 13 Quality Improvement: Quality Improvement and Patient-Centered Care 123

Chapter 14 Just the Beginning 131

Epilogue 139

Index 143

DETAILED CONTENTS

Acknowledgments xv

Prologue xvii

Part I Introduction 1

Chapter 1 Contemplating a Career in Nursing 3

- The Gallup Poll 3
- Environmental Theory: Florence Nightingale 3
- Nursing: Head, Heart, and Hands 4
- The Nursing Process 5
- Evidence-Based Practice (EBP) 7
- EBP and Critical Thinking 8
- Nursing: Scope of Practice 9
- The Leadership Journey in Nursing: Passing the Torch 10
- Lifelong Learning: Continuing Education in Nursing 10
- Current Trends in Nursing 11
- Patient-Centered Care 12
- Investigating Nursing Programs 14
- Reflective Questions 14
- Food for Thought 15
- References 16

Part II Critical Incidents 19

Chapter 2 The Critical Incident: Change 21

- Introduction 21
- Critical Incident One 21
- Critical Incident Two 22
- Change Theory: Kurt Lewin 23
- Reflective Questions 24
- Scenario 25
- Food for Thought 25
- References 26

Chapter 3	Caring	29
	Introduction	29
	Critical Incident One	30
	Critical Incident Two	31
	Reflective Questions	32
	Scenario	32
	Questions	32
	Food for Thought	33
	References	35
Chapter 4	Integrating Theory and Evidence-Based Practice	37
	Introduction	37
	Critical Incident One	38
	Critical Incident Two	39
	Reflective Questions	40
	Scenario	40
	Food for Thought	41
	References	42
Chapter 5	Communication and Culture	43
	Introduction	43
	Cultural Awareness	43
	Critical Incident One	44
	Critical Incident Two	45
	Food for Thought	47
	Forward in Health Medical Mission Trip	50
	Scenario	52
	Reflective Questions	52
	References	52
Chapter 6	Civility	53
	Introduction	53
	Critical Incident One	53
	Critical Incident Two	54
	Reflective Questions	55
	Scenario	56
	Food for Thought	56
	References	57
Chapter 7	Lifelong Learning	59
	Introduction	59
	Critical Incident One	59
	Intuition	61
	Critical Incident Two	61
	Reflective Questions	63
	Introduction to the Scenario	63
	Scenario	64
	Reflection	64
	Food for Thought	64
	References	65

Chapter 8 Resilience 67
Introduction 67
Critical Incident One 67
Critical Incident Two 69
Reflective Questions 70
Scenario 71
Food for Thought 71
References 73

Part III Looking Ahead 75

Chapter 9 Growing Our Own 77
Introduction 77
The Nursing Shortage 78
The Nursing Shortage: Growing Our Own 79
The Nursing Faculty Shortage 80
The Nursing Faculty Shortage: Reversing the Trend Through Mentoring 81
Benefits of a Mentoring Program 83
The Nurse Educator in Academia 83
The Novice Nurse Educator: Orientation to the Faculty Role 84
Implications for Nursing Practice 85
Reflective Questions 85
Scenario 85
Questions for Further Discussion 87
Food for Thought 87
References 89

Chapter 10 Building a Culture of Safety 91
Introduction 91
The Fallout From Incivility 91
Upholding Civility Within the Profession of Nursing 93
The Role of Nursing Leadership in Establishing and Maintaining Civility 94
Learning From Adverse Events 95
Tools Fostering Safety and Civility 96
Finding Balance: Combating Burnout and Compassion Fatigue 96
The Durability of Resilience 97
Reflective Questions 97
Scenario 98
Questions 98
Food for Thought 98
References 100

Chapter 11 Cultural Literacy 103
Introduction 103
Cultural Dissonance 103
Cultural Literacy 104
Leininger's Theory of Culture Care: Diversity and Universality (1991) 104

Cultural Assessment: The "Four C's of Culture" Model 105
Cultivating Cultural Self-Awareness 106
Social Determinants of Health 107
Food Insecurity 108
Healthy People 2030 109
Holism 110
Reflective Questions 111
Scenario 111
Questions to Consider 111
Food for Thought 111
References 113

Chapter 12 Informatics Literacy: Strengthening Informatics and Health Information Literacy 115
Kotter's Model of Change 115
Informatics Technology (IT) Education 116
Telehealth 117
The Use of "Wearables" 117
The Nursing Informatics Specialist (NIS) 118
Reflective Questions 119
Scenario 119
Questions 120
Food for Thought 120
References 121

Chapter 13 Quality Improvement: Quality Improvement and Patient-Centered Care 123
Introduction 123
The Quality Improvement Model 123
The Plan-Do-Study-Act (PDSA) Cycle 124
QI and Root Cause Analysis (RCA) 124
QI and Lewin's Change Theory 125
Benefits of Quality Improvement 125
Reflective Questions 126
Scenario 126
Questions 127
Food for Thought 127
References 129

Chapter 14 Just the Beginning 131
Professional Development and Continuing Education 131
Maintaining the Quality of Patient Care: The New Seven P's of Nursing 132
Expanding the Nursing Pipeline 133
Transition to Practice 134
Reflective Questions 134
Scenario 134
Food for Thought 135
References 136

Epilogue 139
Index 143

ACKNOWLEDGMENTS

Let no one ever come to you without leaving better and happier.

—Mother Teresa

No achievements in life can be accomplished without the support of others. I credit my parents, who believed in education and afforded their children that opportunity; my grandparents, with their kind, quiet ways, who lived with us during our formative years, reinforced family values and ethics, and personified the Golden Rule.

When I became a parent, it was my siblings who were always there, offering unconditional love and support, and to hold me up during personal crisis. It was my husband who supported me upon my return to school, during writing and presenting my research, and becoming a published author of two books. It was my older children who were invaluable in helping us raise their younger brothers. When the older two left for college and beyond, my younger "cheerleaders" kept me young with their "energy." It was a group of my closest friends and nursing colleagues, who lent support, never judged, and were always there to listen. I am indebted to these individuals for contributing to a life and vocation where I feel I made a difference. Finally, I credit my longevity in nursing education to my students—my greatest teachers.

Growing up as a clumsy tomboy, I experienced many fractured bones and spent a lot of time in the emergency department, where I first learned to understand the vital role of nurses. Since the age of 4, I have always wanted to work in healthcare in some way. This led to my working as a nurse's aide in high school and college, where I met and admired a multitude of nursing role models. After graduation, my first nursing job was "floating" to different units working nights in the hospital. This was an invaluable chance to experience where in the profession I wanted to practice (and where I did not). As a pediatric nurse, I happened to meet a nursing professor whose children were often hospitalized, who convinced me to try my hand at clinical instruction. I became immediately "hooked."

Becoming a nurse educator, however, required a return to academia after 13 years of clinical nursing practice. I was initially intimidated, but with the support of qualified, informed educators, friendly and smart classmates, and cheered on by fellow nursing colleagues I survived. I recognized the importance of the courses studied and saw how the concepts applied to my nursing practice. Education opened doors for me.

PROLOGUE

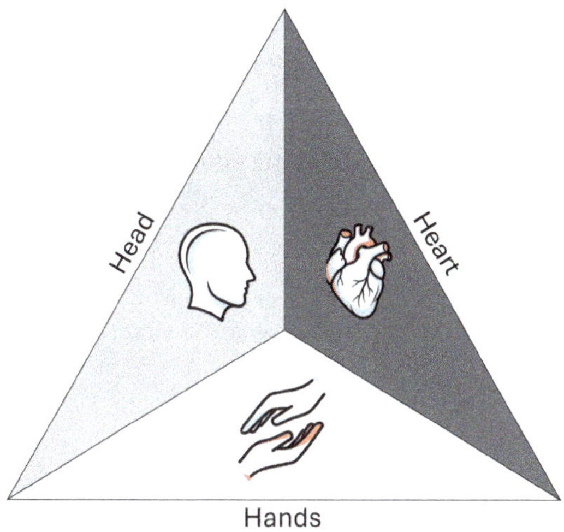

Figure P.1 Head, Heart, and Hands
Created by Brian Duphily

We learn from one another how to be human by identifying ourselves with others, finding their dilemmas in ourselves. What we all learn from it is self-knowledge. The self we learn about is every self. It is universal -the human self. We learn to recognize ourselves in others.

(Watson 1985)

Purpose

This work is not your conventional textbook. There are no lesson plans, specific objectives, quizzes, adaptive test questions, abstract professional concepts, or games. Included are reflection activities, scenarios, historical concepts, nursing theories, however. *Head, Heart, and Hands* is much more than the above content often requires in textbooks. It is written for nurses, students, parents of students, individuals considering a career in (or a career change to) nursing, and for the general public, who wonder what it is that nurses actually "do", and how they are prepared for this role. Through dissemination of nurses' stories, it is this author's intent to carry nurses' voices and to celebrate the cognitive, affective, and psychomotor ("head, heart, and hands") skills nurses employ on a daily basis with each of their patients, regardless of setting, specialty, or patient population.

My hope is that the reader will gain a better understanding of the multifaceted nature of the nursing profession, how educators and mentors prepare and "grow" nurses throughout their career, and what strategies nurses employ on a daily basis with the societal, environmental and physical demands placed on nurse's shoulders. In the following pages, through the presentation of shared critical incidents, nursing theories, current challenges, and achievements, I hope to accomplish this task.

Chapters will include the following:

- Nursing figures who came before us and on whose shoulders we stand
- Critical thinking and evidence-based practice
- Application of nursing theories that guide nurse's decision-making
- Significance of mentors throughout a nurse's career
- The educational and clinical preparation of a nursing student
- Struggles nurses face in today's society (i.e., staffing ratios, workplace violence, environmental safety)
- The importance of collaboration with patients, families, and other health care providers
- The necessity of lifelong learning: continuing education in the profession

The Value of Mentoring

Education is the most powerful weapon which you can use to change the world.

—Nelson Mandela

As a nurse and nursing instructor, I have worked and taught in various clinical and educational settings for many years. I received nursing degrees from the University of Massachusetts, Amherst, and have a doctorate of nursing practice (DNP) from Regis College. I came to academia after 13 years in the "real world" of clinical practice. In the academic setting, I found a community of mentors and colleagues who excelled in teaching, nurturing, and guiding others. Teaching has made me a better nurse. It has challenged me to articulate my practice and answer the question "why?" when working with students in both classroom and clinical settings. To nurture and encourage a behavior performed correctly is powerful. The educator that I am today is a result of the careful mentoring of past advisors and current coworkers, along with the thoughtful criticism by my students.

Teaching has afforded me some of my greatest rewards and most significant challenges. It is a skill that requires continuous and ongoing feedback, introspection, and improvement. When I am at my best as a teacher and mentor, I ask and hear what my students need from me and am able to respond appropriately. Each student, class, and clinical group is different. I seek to continually improve my teaching by reaching out to, and receiving honest feedback from, my students and by watching and learning from the many dynamic faculty that surround me daily. Empowering students to acknowledge, value, and apply the principles of the requisite liberal arts and sciences courses as part of their nursing education provides them with the intellectual tools and background needed for a career of lifelong learning and continued growth in the profession. In my educational journey, I have been fortunate to have exceptional mentors each step of the way. Mentoring, however, does not subscribe to the "one-size-fits-all" approach, nor does it assume one particular identity in an individual.

Looking back, I recognize and appreciate those benevolent, informal mentors who took the time to review my "work in progress": paper corrections, test construction, advice with student problems, and clinical challenges. As painful sometimes as it was to hear their frank feedback, I learned from the best. They valued their mentoring role and took the job of guiding the next generation of educators seriously. I was advised to sit in on other faculty's lectures and in time learned to develop my own eclectic style and to hone my craft. At times, I felt like I was a mere breath ahead of my students, nontraditional learners, human sponges. They demanded their education and had fought many internal, personal battles to win a coveted seat in nursing class. I grew to love every minute of it.

I recognized the importance of mentorship as I began to consider pursuing further advanced practice in nursing education, when asked by my dean if I might be interested in teaching a part-time course in a local university's nurse educator program. The director of this program met with me at the beginning of the course to outline the curriculum she had developed. She was always there for me throughout the semester. As I taught the course, I remember wishing that I had completed such an educational program 20 years before. In essence, this educational experience provided those contemplating a career in nursing education the courage to make this daunting role transition.

Weekly topics included test construction, legal aspects, ethical dilemmas, student issues, and creation of syllabi. I discovered that I was never able to get through all of the material. My students were new educators in need of a forum to vent their feelings, experiences, and challenges. Much of their dialogue revolved around the fact that there was "no one to go to" with problems. The discussions were lively, fascinating, sometimes quite heated, but never dull. I looked forward to the weekly debates. The lesson plan sometimes took a detour. I came to realize the importance of this exchange of ideas. It bonded this class quite uniquely. More importantly, it inspired me to return to academia for my DNP.

Fifty years later, I continue to learn each day. As an adjunct faculty member in the RN to BS in Nursing Program of a local university, I teach an online course to approximately 40 students each semester. The students enrolled in this course are typically associate degree in nursing (ADN) graduates who wish to advance their education in order to become leaders in their workplace or secure employment in the acute care hospital setting. They are articulate, open, and engaged. As the course typically requires these students to "apply theory to practice," they share many stories, supporting these assignments, about their current experience as nurses. Some students are novices, having recently graduated from entry level nursing education; others are veteran nurses, required by their employers to return to academia for a baccalaureate degree (BSN) to maintain their current position or to climb the leadership ladder.

Some are not always happy to return. I have made it a point to welcome their experience, education, and expertise by asking them to share their career history on the discussion board and by celebrating publicly the value they bring to the academic "table." This reception not only encourages sharing among students but opens the door for mutual collegial support in their common pursuit of the BSN degree. As *Transitions* is the initial course in the RN to BS program, it is incumbent upon me as their instructor to set the stage of expectations and to foster their collegiality as they navigate through and complete each class toward their baccalaureate degree goal.

In the past 5 years (2020–2025), students' "critical incidents" have focused on the COVID-19 pandemic and its fallout. They relate poignant, heartbreaking stories of their struggles as nurses, working with scarce supplies and staff, being sole caregivers holding the hands of dying patients whose loved ones were not permitted on the unit, and returning home to their families, worrying all the while if they were infecting their loved ones with this unknown disease that was taking away the lives of their patients.

Other stories students shared involved those who were nursing students during COVID, the domino effect it had on their education, and, ultimately, on their practice as graduate nurses. This cohort had to adjust and adapt to delays and cancellations, remote lectures, and simulation methodology as a significant component of their education and clinical experience. They were filled with gratitude to their hard-working and creative nursing educators for the improvised education they were receiving. Years later, many now cite the difficulties they experienced as new graduates, citing that they often left their first nursing position, reporting overwhelming feelings of inadequacy.

The series of events that transpired following the March 2020 COVID pandemic produced many new and conflicting emotions, from anxiety, disbelief, and terror, to sadness, hope, and optimism. In "remote" conversations with friends, relatives, colleagues, and students, it was apparent that many shared similar conflicting emotions during this crisis—emotions that appeared to change on a daily basis. We found which strategies helped weather the storm and those that did not.

Communicating the stories of nurses, both past and present, celebrating their daily workplace challenges and victories, and acknowledging the contributions being brought to the academic table are the primary messages I hope to convey to readers. Nurses demonstrate the remarkable ability to support others during their own individual periods of vulnerability. To risk peril in their work on a daily basis demands an uncommon degree of selflessness and bravery.

Accounts of nurses' struggles and their commitment during the COVID-19 pandemic inspired me to create this book, a compilation of the accomplishments nurses perform each day. I am honored to be part of such a profession, one which afforded me the opportunity to be a part of some of the most intimate moments in people's lives, to experience lifelong learning, to raise a family and provide a good life for my children, and to this day, to maintain friendships and alliances with an incredible group of like-minded, ethical, empathetic, and supportive people who are still my friends today.

Moreover, I wish to educate the public about nurses, these "lifelong students," many of whom are practicing today under extreme circumstances, returning each day to repeat the same work, all while caring for family members, all still finding time to return to school. Too, they find time to express their gratitude for online education; for many, it was the only way to return to school.

The nurses featured in this book share powerful, poignant, and valuable insights related to caring for patients across diverse ages, cultures, and backgrounds. They have it right. It is time that the public knew what it takes to become (and to stay) a nurse.

Equally important for the reader to understand is what it takes to "grow a nurse." What is involved in this mentoring process of producing a graduate who is responsible for the lives of others? Incorporating the perspective of nurse educators is key in the future preparation and advancement of nurses for the challenges of a new generation. The role of the nurse educator is not clearly defined. It is often a true baptism-by-fire experience. With veteran instructors retiring at an alarming rate, how do we attract practicing nurses to the educator role?

Figure Credit

Fig. P.1: Generated using Google Gemini.

PART I

1 Introduction

CHAPTER 1

Contemplating a Career in Nursing

What you do makes a difference.

You have to decide what kind of difference you want to make.

—Jane Goodall

The Gallup Poll

Regardless of the daily challenges they face, nurses have been recognized annually for the key role they play in maintaining the health and safety of the nation. The Gallup Poll rating illustrates that nurses generate a significant and positive impact in the health care system. With a response of 78%, the nursing profession was ranked as the most trusted profession for the 21st year in a row. This recognition belongs to America's nurses, who continue to navigate through a challenging and ongoing nursing shortage (Saad, 2025).

As the largest segment of caregivers in the health care workforce, nurses are the primary providers of hospitalized patient care and deliver most of the nation's long-term care. With the nursing profession numbers projected to increase by 5% from 2021 to 2031, growth in the RN workforce is centered on the emphasis of preventive care, an increase in chronic conditions, and the burgeoning need for health care services from the baby-boom population (American Association of Colleges of Nursing [AACN], 2022).

Employers are expressing a strong preference for new nurses with baccalaureate preparation. Findings from the *Employment of New Nurse Graduates Survey* (AACN, 2022) show that nearly 28% of employers require new hires to have a bachelor's degree, while 72% prefer baccalaureate-prepared nurses. In 2022, 17.4% of the nation's registered nurses possessed a master's degree; 2.7% possessed a doctoral degree as their highest educational preparation. The current demand for master's- and doctorally prepared nurses for advanced practice, clinical specialties, teaching, and research roles far surpasses the current supply (Smiley et al., 2023)

Environmental Theory: Florence Nightingale

Possessing an evidence-based practice philosophy was initiated through the work and influence of nurse Florence Nightingale and her environmental theory model. Working overseas as a nursing supervisor in a military hospital during the Crimean War (1853–1856), Nightingale used critical thinking skills and judgment to determine how the environment influenced patient health. Nightingale chronicled her findings in the groundbreaking book *Notes on Nursing* (Karimi & Masoudi, 2015).

The events of the Civil War (1861–1865) demonstrated the need for experienced health providers, particularly for women. Before this time, women functioned in the caregiver role as private duty nurses, guided by years of experience tending to the needs of family members rather than by designated, official training centers. In 1861, there were no organized field hospital services or training services for medical assistance on the battlefield. The title "nurse" could refer to a woman appointed by the superintendent of women nurses for the Union Army, an officer's wife, mothers caring for a wounded son or husband who stayed on to care for others, or "camp followers" (Culpepper & Adams, 1988).

The Civil War highlighted the need for formal nursing education for practice. At this same time, Nightingale had become a well-known public figure in England, with her forceful support of women in the role as capable professionals. In 1872, Nightingale's work was replicated in the United States with the establishment of the New England Hospital for Women and Children, a formal nurse training program that shared similar principles to the ones Nightingale had established. Within a year, three "Nightingale schools" opened in America: the New York Training School at Bellevue Hospital, the Connecticut Training School at New Haven Hospital, and the Boston Training School at Massachusetts General Hospital. Her published works *Notes on Nursing* (1859) and *Notes on Hospitals* (1859) impacted American audiences to the extent that nurses in the Civil War were referred to as "Nightingales." Throughout the Civil War, Nightingale was frequently consulted about how to best manage field hospitals (Karimi & Masoudi, 2015).

Nursing: Head, Heart, and Hands

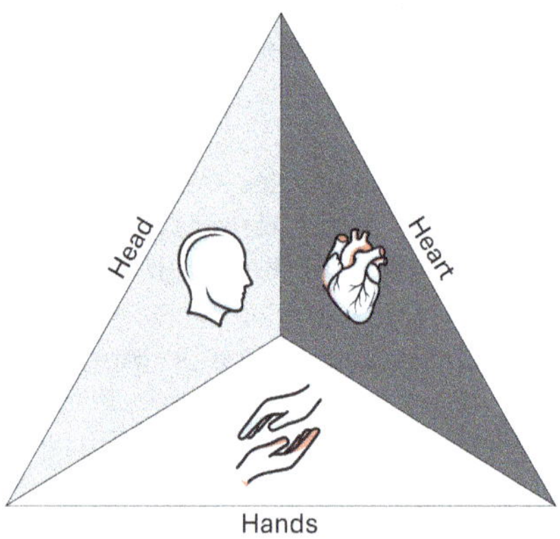

Figure 1.1 Head, Heart, and Hands
Created by Brian Duphily

Wherever there is someone in need of care, nurses are present, working diligently to identify and attend to the needs of patients. Behind a strong reputation for empathy, caring, and commitment lies a highly specialized professional. The key unifying characteristic in every role in the profession is the skill and drive that it takes to be a nurse. The journey of a demanding entry-level nursing program, years of clinical experience honing their craft and expertise, continuing education, a keenly developed sense of intuition, and strong patient advocacy skills, places nurses in a reliable position to weigh in on a patient's well-being. Daily, nurses use cognitive, affective, and psychomotor skills ("head, heart, and hands") in their work, to adapt, learn and evolve, in addressing the dynamic nature of healthcare (Sipos et al., 2008).

The "head" (cognitive) involves creating, promoting, and providing a plan of evidence-based care, anticipating resistance, and strategizing to resolve related issues. It includes listening to patients and collaborating with colleagues to better understand and communicate to others a proposed intervention and its expected outcome (Shaikh & Lachman, 2021).

> *The best and most beautiful things in the world cannot be seen or even touched.*
>
> *They must be felt with the heart.*
>
> *—Helen Keller*

The "heart" (affective) refers to those human, emotional aspects of planning an intervention. This involves calling on one's incentive, personal goals, and values. Anticipating resistance is a key consideration here, as engaging the heart involves building trust and developing a climate of psychological safety where those who question a plan are heard. Communication strategies to engage the heart should include patient and provider narratives "to demonstrate the benefits of the innovation and the consequences of not changing" (Shaikh & Lachman, 2021, p. 2).

The "hands" (psychomotor) refers to carrying out the plan. The actions of the nurse in this area convey a clear connection between the interventions and the future state. It involves tracking progress, identifying goals achieved, and gathering support. Communication strategies here include pointing out the benefits of the intervention and its outcome with patients and fellow providers (Shaikh & Lachman, 2021).

The Nursing Process

Assessment, Diagnosis, Planning, Implementation, Evaluation (ADPIE)

Complementing the "head, heart, and hands" philosophy is the "nursing process," a scientific, five-step method designed to deliver informed, holistic, and comprehensive nursing care to all patient populations. Through the "critical thinking" method represented in the steps of the nursing process, nurses use their judgment to integrate objective data with the subjective experience of a patient's biological, physical, and behavioral needs (Lofti et al., 2021).

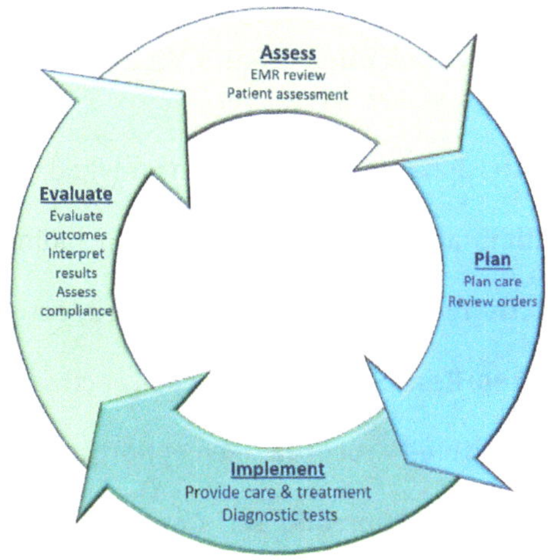

Figure 1.2 Nursing Process: Assess, Plan, Implement, Evaluate

- **Assessment:** the nurse completes a comprehensive patient examination to identify the patient's current and future care needs, develop an individualized care plan, and provide appropriate interventions. Patient assessment data typically includes the following: chief complaint, physical and psychosocial examination, vital signs measurements, and biographical, social, health, and medication histories.
- **Diagnosis:** the nurse forms a **"nursing diagnosis**," the "human response" to the medical diagnosis, through careful consideration of both physical symptoms and patient behavior. After analyzing the data and determining relevant cues, the nurse clusters data into patterns. Assessment frameworks such as Gordon's functional health patterns (see next) assist nurses in clustering information according to evidence-based patterns of human responses. The functional health patterns (FHP) model created by Marjory Gordon continues as a valuable nursing tool (Hiriscau et al., 2024). It presents an all-inclusive, organized, and systematic means to assess human functioning. Gordon's methodology guides nurses to examine and identify evidence related to health, illness, and nursing care. From the data collected, nurses create a problem statement and a **"nursing diagnosis," the "human response" to the physician's medical diagnosis.** For example, the patient with a medical diagnosis of stroke who is experiencing paralysis would lead the nurse to identify a human response/nursing diagnosis as "impaired skin integrity." The nurse selects

this "problem" from a list of the North American Nursing Diagnosis Association's (NANDA) approved nursing diagnoses in developing a prioritized, individualized nursing care plan (Carpenito, 2017).

Gordon's Functional Health Patterns

Marjory Gordon's functional health patterns provide a structured way to conduct an organized, comprehensive, holistic patient assessment (Gordon, 1994). The FHP approach supports the myriad of human responses to the medical diagnosis and fosters deeper diagnostic reasoning. This framework enables nurses the ability to collect data, identify patterns, and form nursing diagnoses across biological, social, and spiritual dimensions.

Health Perception–Health Management: A patient's perception of their health and well-being and how it is managed

Nutritional-Metabolic: Food and fluid consumption relative to metabolic need

Elimination: Excretory function, including bowel, bladder, and skin

Activity-Exercise: Exercise and daily activities

Sleep-Rest: Sleep, rest, and daily activities

Cognitive-Perceptual: Perception and cognition

Self-Perception and Self-Concept: Self-concept and perception of self-worth, self-competency, body image, and mood state

Role-Relationship: Role engagements and relationships

Sexuality-Reproductive: Reproduction and satisfaction or dissatisfaction with sexuality

Coping-Stress Tolerance: Coping and effectiveness in terms of stress tolerance

Value-Belief: Values, beliefs (including spiritual beliefs), and goals that guide choices and decisions

- **Outcomes/Planning:** The nurse sets realistic goals for the patient's recovery with the patient. Goals are guided by the "SMART" mnemonic: specific, measurable, attainable, realistic, and time oriented.
- **Implementation:** The nurse carries out and documents the plan, guaranteeing consistency of care for the patient. Nursing rationales are often included to provide the reasoning behind specific actions taken in patient care. They are grounded in evidence-based practice and tailored to the patient's individual needs.
- **Evaluation:** By closely analyzing the effectiveness of the care plan and studying patient response, the nurse hones the plan to achieve the very best patient outcomes. Ideally, when the planned interventions are implemented, the patient will respond positively, and the expected outcomes are achieved. However, when interventions do not assist in progressing the patient toward the expected outcomes, the nursing care plan must be revised to more effectively address the needs of the patient (Toney-Butler & Thayer, 2023).

The nursing process is fluid and dynamic. It changes with the patient response to the care plan initiated. The needs of the patient may shift, problems may resolve, or new issues may surface. The following questions can be used as a guide when revising the nursing care plan:

- Did anything unanticipated occur?
- Has the patient's condition changed?
- Were the expected outcomes and their time frames realistic?
- Are the nursing diagnoses accurate for this patient at this time?
- Are the planned interventions appropriately focused on supporting outcome attainment?
- What barriers were experienced as interventions were implemented?
- Does ongoing assessment data indicate the need to revise diagnoses, outcome criteria, planned interventions, or implementation strategies?
- Are different interventions required?

Critical thinking is used throughout the nursing process continually when assessing the patient, creating a nursing care plan, and implementing interventions. Reassessment and revisions to the care plan are adjusted in assisting the patient to achieve expected outcomes. Throughout the cyclical nursing process, the patient is not only the focus of nursing care but functions in the role of an active participant in the plan, if possible.

These are the steps of **ADPIE**. These components involve assessing, planning, and providing individualized, patient-centered care. Nurses evaluate whether that care has been successful in achieving patient outcomes and return to the plan to adjust goals. These objectives are essential for professional nursing practice in providing safe, current, and informed patient care (Toney-Butler & Thayer, 2023).

Evidence-Based Practice (EBP)

Intellectual growth should commence at birth and cease only at death.

—Albert Einstein

Considered the "father" of evidenced-based medicine (EBM), Dr. Archibald Cochrane (1909–1988) voiced his concern regarding the lack of scientific evidence substantiating medical interventions. Heightened by his own experiences as a practicing physician attempting to cure tuberculosis, he worried that he actually might be doing more harm than good for these individuals (Shah & Chung, 2009).

Cochrane believed that existing medical interventions based on assumptions led to inconsistencies in the delivery of care. He theorized that health care delivery should be based on procedures proven to be most effective (Mackey & Bassendowski, 2017). No medical intervention should be performed without evidence validating its effectiveness; instead, a systematic and scientifically based approach to the clinical practice of medicine should direct all clinical decisions. The concepts he formulated, in particular the requirement of random controlled trials (RCTs) to determine the appropriate treatment, and the importance of examining cost-effectiveness, created a significant impact on clinical medicine.

Cochrane's 1971 publication "Effectiveness and Efficiency" criticized the lack of reliable evidence for health care practices during this period of time. His concerns prompted precise appraisal of health care practices in the search for accurate evidence in medicine (Shah & Chung, 2009). Five years after his death, his efforts to require an evidence-supporting practice resulted in the development of the Cochrane Collaboration. This international organization produces quality, up-to-date systematic reviews and information related to outcomes of different treatments.

EBM is described today as a formal practice of decision-making based on the best treatment practice of patient from a systematic detailed method of research evidence. "Evidence-based medicine" was subsequently retitled "evidence-based practice," given its use as a practice standard across multiple disciplines (Mackey & Bassendowski, 2017).

For nurses, EBP challenges nurses to expand their knowledge base and standardizes best nursing practices (Abu-Baker et al., 2021) Fundamental to nursing, it allows nurses to understand diagnoses, treatments, and procedures. This philosophy supports nurses in their understanding of the reasons for performing care, and how these actions influence patient outcomes.

EBP and Critical Thinking

Critical thinking, clinical reasoning, and judgment are all essential in developing EBP guidelines in nursing care. Critical thinking and reasoning require the evaluation of disease processes and nursing practices to improve patient care. They allow nurses to think outside of the box, beyond the current standards of practice. Critical thinking aids in the development of new policies and procedures. The ability to reason and have judgment can help nurses have an open mind and evaluate current standards. A nurse with an open mind will critique current practices to ensure that they are accurate and meet patient needs. A nurse who is close minded will not evaluate the current practice and will continue the practice even if it is not accurate and does not meet patient needs (McGrath, 2005).

Critical thinking and reasoning are also important because they allow nurses to plan their interventions prior to implementation. This allows nurses to assess the situation and evaluate the standard of care before providing care. If there was ever a discrepancy or outdated policy, this would give nurses the ability to rectify that discrepancy. Without critical thinking, there would be more room for error and poorer patient health outcomes.

The process of EBP in nursing follows a structured, step-by-step approach to ensure the effective application of research into clinical practice. The first step involves formulating a clear clinical question, often framed using the PICOT approach, which stands for *patient/population, intervention, comparison, outcome,* and *time*. The second step involves searching for the best available evidence through reliable databases, clinical guidelines, and peer-reviewed studies. After gathering data from research, the third step is selecting relevant studies, where nurses evaluate the quality, validity, and relevance of the research. After determining the most credible evidence, the fourth step is integrating the evidence with clinical expertise and patient preferences to guide decision-making (Bell, 2020). Finally, the fifth step is evaluating measurable outcomes of the intervention. The process concludes with dissemination of findings and applying lessons learned to future nursing practice, contributing to the improvement of patient care.

An important factor in successful implementation of EBP into practice is creating a culture of willingness to change within health care institutions (Bell, 2020). This involves encouraging nurses to question traditional practices, seek out new evidence, and be open to integrating research into their daily routines. Leadership skills play an important role by promoting EBP, offering resources, and supporting initiatives that prioritize evidence-based decision-making. As the nursing profession continues to evolve, implementing EBP remains crucial in addressing new challenges, improving health care delivery, and ensuring that nursing practice remains at the forefront of innovation and excellence.

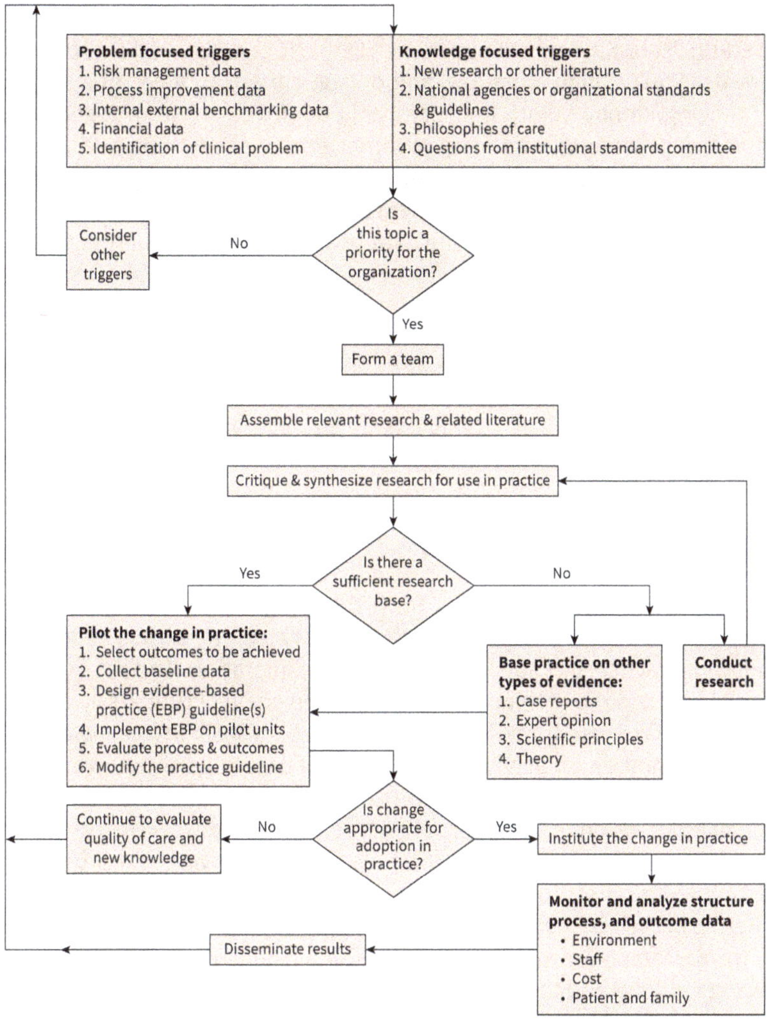

Figure 1.3 The Iowa Model of Evidence-Based Practice to Promote Quality Care

Nursing: Scope of Practice

> *Nursing integrates the art and science of caring and focuses on the protection, promotion, and optimization of health and human functioning; prevention of illness and injury; facilitation of healing; and alleviation of suffering through compassionate presence. Nursing is the diagnosis and treatment of human responses and advocacy in the care of individuals, families, groups, communities, and populations in recognition of the connection of all humanity.*
>
> *(ANA, 2021, p. 1)*

From the above ANA (2021) definition, it is evident that nurses work diligently to recognize and protect the needs of their patients. Educated, experienced nurses use specialized, diverse skills to address the needs of current society. Nurses play a crucial role in achieving safe, effective, and holistic care of patients. Nurses save lives. A registered nurse has obtained a nursing degree, passed the National Council Licensure Exam (NCLEX-RN), and completed state licensing requirements. Nurses align, organize, and deliver care in all areas of a patient's health. A patient experiencing kidney failure may seek collaborative care from a general practitioner, cardiologist, and nephrologist, who work together to diagnose, treat, and prescribe medications based on their area of expertise. The nurse is responsible for overseeing the patient's full care, ensuring that medications and treatments prescribed for the patient do not negatively interact with one another, verifying that the patient understands and agrees to comply with the care plan.

The Leadership Journey in Nursing: Passing the Torch

Rejoice in your work; never lose sight of the nursing leader you are now and the nursing leader you will become.

—Sue Fitzsimons, PhD, RN, CNO at Yale–New Haven

The "passing the torch" metaphor stems from the ancient Greek torch relay race, where a lighted torch was passed from one runner to the next. It involves leaders' relinquishing responsibilities, tradition, practice, or knowledge to the next generation. The act symbolized the passage of responsibility and the continuity of an unbroken chain of runners. In a broader context, this phrase is used to represent the act of passing on responsibility, knowledge, or authority from one person to another, often with the intention of ensuring continuity and success.

The passing of the torch is an ongoing process to identify and develop the talent flourishing in the nursing profession (Chichester, 2009). Identifying leaders early in their career is key to success, satisfaction, and longevity in the role. In turn, growing and producing great leaders sets an example for others to follow. They live out the core values of the organization, and they are authentic in their pursuit of growth. They view learning as a lifelong process, and they invite others to grow and learn along the way by sharing and investing in the growth of others.

Great leaders understand their place in the line of generational leadership. They are grateful for the incredible leaders who have come before them and invested in their lives, and they demonstrate their appreciation by investing in future generations of leaders. The biggest "thank you" they can give to past mentors is to pass these lessons on to future mentees.

Lifelong Learning: Continuing Education in Nursing

Nursing is an art: and if it is to be made an art, it requires an exclusive devotion as hard a preparation as any painter's or sculptor's work.

—Florence Nightingale

Continuing education units (CEUs) in nursing include nursing education beyond what is required for entry-level practice. CEUs allow nurses to build upon their education and experience, develop their abilities and knowledge, maintain nursing credentials and a nursing license, and continue their practice in a clinical setting. Advances in medical technology, medications, and treatments are ever changing in healthcare. Continuing nursing education provides the opportunity to learn about new treatment strategies or new indications for existing treatment that can help provide patients with the best care available. With CEUs, nurses are able to refine existing knowledge and advance their nursing skills in order to support "best practices" in the workplace (ANA, 2015).

Requirements for nursing continuing education (CE) differ according to each state's board of nursing. Some states require a specific number of contact hours for licensure, while other states require that both CE hours and specific CE course topics are completed as part of the license renewal process. A contact hour is defined as the "unit" awarded for a nurse's participation in CE (ANA, 2021). Satisfying CE requirements advances knowledge and skills. It carries the potential for advancing one's position and corresponds with a higher salary. Additionally, CE demonstrates dedication to the profession. This knowledge contributes to the performance of job responsibilities with greater confidence and assurance, ultimately leading to greater job satisfaction and improving the care patients receive. Finally, CE is essential in the development of informed nurses to assume the role of mentors. Continuing nursing education, whether presented remotely (webinars), face-to-face classes, seminars, or skills fairs, enables advancing one's knowledge and position as a trusted resource and leader in the workplace (Harper & Maloney, 2022).

Current Trends in Nursing

Delivery of health services in dynamic and challenging environments calls for nurses who must continually learn and grow to guarantee quality, informed patient care. Staying ahead of emerging trends is not only a professional obligation but also a necessary requirement for maintaining patient safety. Technological advances, societal shifts, and evolving health care needs significantly impact daily nursing practice among all workplace settings, calling for adaptability to change, along with a proactive approach to professional growth.

The nursing profession is at a pivotal juncture. By embracing new technologies, developing new skills, and advocating for policies that support quality patient care, nurses can continue to significantly contribute to the health and well-being of individuals and communities. Continuous learning and adaptation are essential for navigating the complexities of the evolving health care landscape. By staying informed about emerging trends, nurses can ensure they are well-equipped to meet future challenges.

Integration of Technology

Telehealth and remote patient communication are prevalent, enabling nurses to provide care beyond the traditional hospital setting. Virtual consultations, remote monitoring of vital signs, and home-based care programs enhance patient access while improving efficiency. Wearable technology is gaining traction in patient care. Smartwatches, fitness trackers, and other wearable devices can collect valuable patient data, such as heart rate, activity levels, and sleep patterns. This data can be utilized to monitor patient health, identify potential risks, and personalize care plans.

Artificial Intelligence (AI) in Healthcare

AI has impacted health care delivery practices with the integration of systematic algorithms, or steps, to assist with patient diagnosis and treatment planning, as well as scheduling and documentation responsibilities. Conveying the AI "selling points" of improving time and accuracy has the potential for creating a more efficient and effective health care environment.

In "Prediction to Practice: AI's Role in Healthcare 2025," *Forbes* member Greg Samios (2025) writes, "The priority is ensuring that providers receive the right information, in the right channels, at the right time." Providers prioritize speed in receiving accurate data as key to producing positive health care outcomes for patients. Confirming, too, that the correct information is obtained, effectively increases the impact of clinical decision support (Samios, 2025).

"Point-of-care GenAI" places generative artificial intelligence (GenAI) directly at the location where a patient is being treated. Benefits include immediate access to information and location flexibility. Equipped with tablets and smartphones, nurses and other health professionals can readily access AI capabilities at the patient's bedside (Samios, 2025).

Recognition of the benefits of AI in healthcare depends on providers' involvement and investment in the technology, as well as their understanding and perseverance in addressing those areas of concern needing attention and resolution. Patients' approval and participation are crucial elements in building trust with the technology. Active clinician participation in the system, when articulated to patients, has the potential to positively impact acceptance and support of AI.

Patient-Centered Care

I think health care is more about love than about most other things. If there isn't love at the core, with two human beings who have agreed to be in a relationship, where one is trying to help relieve the suffering of another, you can't get to the right answer here.

—Donald Berwick, MD, former administrator of the Centers for Medicare and Medicaid

In 1986, businessman, educator, inventor, and philanthropist Dr. Harvey Picker founded the Boston-based Picker Institute, a not-for-profit organization dedicated to developing a patient-centered approach to healthcare. Dr. Picker believed that the American health care system was technologically and scientifically outstanding. Glaringly absent, he felt, was the overall responsiveness to patients' concerns and comfort levels.

Over the course of seven years, Picker and his team interviewed more than 8,000 patients, family members, physicians, and hospital staff about their personal interactions with the health care system. Findings indicated that patients lacked a trusting relationship with their providers, received insufficient information about their care, and experienced poor communication between themselves and their health care providers. These themes became the foundation for the Picker Survey, the first-ever patient-centered performance measurement tool. This initiative led to the coining of the term **patient-centered care**. With the development of the first scientifically validated patient-experience survey, patients' interactions with the health care delivery system were documented, culminating in the following Principles of Patient-Centered Care (Picker Institute, 2013b):

1. ***Respect for Patients' Values, Preferences, and Expressed Needs.*** All health care providers must involve patients in decision-making, acknowledging that they possess distinct values and preferences. Providers need to demonstrate empathy, respect, and sensitivity related to patients' cultural values and independence
2. ***Coordination and Integration of Care.*** Patients cited feelings of vulnerability and helplessness during their illnesses. Collaboration among providers invested in the plan of care can significantly improve the patient experience. Patients recognized that coordination of clinical care and ancillary and support services can impact communication and reduce feelings of vulnerability.

3. ***Information and Education.*** Patients interviewed revealed they felt uninformed regarding their conditions, diagnoses, and prognoses. By involving patients in discussions about their clinical status, their progress and prognosis, providers can inspire patients' autonomy as well as compliance with treatment.
4. ***Physical Comfort.*** Patients reported that achieving physical comfort significantly affected their hospital experience. Pain management was linked to the level of assistance needed with activities in the hospital environment and surroundings (such as patient transfer to x-ray, physical and occupational therapy).
5. ***Emotional support and alleviation of fear and anxiety.*** The impact of illness on patients and their families, coupled with loss of employment and subsequent financial burdens, are major stressors during hospitalization. The continual emotional support and collaboration of the health care provider team with the patient and family can significantly reduce fears related to patient diagnosis, plan of care, treatments, and prognosis.
6. ***Involvement of Family and Friends.*** Patients recognized family involvement as key in providing patient-centered care. Providing accommodations for family, involving family in decision-making and recognizing and supporting the needs of caregivers are all important elements of this principle.
7. ***Continuity and Transition.*** Patients related concerns post discharge regarding self-care. Providers and health care organizations can assist here by ensuring that detailed information regarding home care, (to include medications, physical limitations, home environment barriers, dietary needs, community resources, and support services) is in place.
8. ***Access to Care.*** Patients expressed the importance of knowing how to access care when needed. Their health care literacy needs included transportation, physical access to health care organizations/clinics, guidance with the ability to schedule office visits and information on scheduling referral appointments.

Patient-centered care continues to prevail as a major focus for providers. In creating an individualized plan based on patients' specific characteristics (i.e., culture, genetics, lifestyle, environmental factors), nurses rely on honed assessment, communication, and interpersonal nursing skills. This approach recognizes and prioritizes patients' unique needs, respects their backgrounds, opinions, and preferences, and ultimately leads to compliance with and active participation in the plan of care.

More than ever, the patient experience is recognized today as a critical factor in health care quality. Beyond clinical outcomes, patient satisfaction, communication, and emotional support significantly influence overall experiences. Nurses play a crucial role in fostering positive patient relationships, addressing concerns, and providing compassionate care. Shared decision-making empowers patients by actively involving them in health care decisions. Nurses facilitate this process by providing clear and unbiased information, addressing patient concerns, and supporting their informed choices (Picker Institute, 2013a, 2013b).

Despite the history of, and widespread attention to, patient-centered care, meaningful engagement with patients continues to be a challenge. Many organizations are still doing things *to* or *for* patients and their families instead of partnering with them. A patient-centered, health care structure strengthens relationships among patients, their families, and their providers. With this type of communication, patients should always know where to go and which individuals to approach to have their questions or concerns addressed. Patient engagement should extend to relationships among staff. Ultimately, if staff members are not interacting effectively with one another, or feel unsupported by the administration, the staff-patient relationship will not prosper.

Effective measurement of patient-centered care is daunting. While the Hospital Consumer Assessment of Healthcare Providers and Systems provides nationally standardized comparative information, it does not measure those issues important to patients and families. Qualitative feedback from patients is detailed and valuable, but many health care organizations struggle with how to use this data effectively to monitor and measure performance. Listening to patients' stories creates the rigor with qualitative metrics that health providers need to improve the patient experience (Picker Institute, 2013a).

Investigating Nursing Programs

You may already have begun to consider if nursing may be **for** you; the next step is to determine which nursing program is of interest **to** you. From this point, take the time to schedule a day to attend a particular college or university program's information session. Tour guides and department officials answer general questions such as scholarship and financial aid, meal plans, academic support, technology services, emergency response protocols, housing options, medical care, counseling, and extracurricular activities.

As a potential nursing major, make sure to take advantage of tours offered by the nursing department, of their classrooms, laboratory, and simulation spaces. Many tours include viewing a simulation activity, conducted by nursing faculty, with current nursing students as participants. Discussion forums are typically held at the end of the tour and are conducted by current nursing students and/or nursing faculty. Questions from the audience usually center on clinical site locations and transportation to these sites, typical class sizes, ratio of clinical faculty to nursing students, and faculty clinical specialties and research interests. Crucial information to obtain from this experience is the nursing program's approval by the Accreditation Commission for Education in Nursing, as well as the yearly percentage of nursing graduates who have successfully passed the National Council Licensure Examination for RNs (NCLEX). The "gold standard" of accreditation is necessary in order for a nursing graduate to take the National Council Licensure Examination (NCLEX) in order to obtain a nursing license.

As you continue on through these chapters, you will come to find that the "head, heart and hands" philosophy of nursing care championed here provides one with the opportunity of a lifelong career of making a difference. This role incorporates so much more than acquiring skills and completing tasks. Hopefully, you will discover that making a difference in someone's life encompasses an unexpected, sometimes overwhelming bumpy terrain. Guaranteed, you will never be bored, you will learn something every day, and you will walk away with vivid memories of your time doing this work.

Opportunities for making a difference range from supporting patients during turbulent or catastrophic times in their lives, counseling patients following a devastating diagnosis, celebrating positive health outcomes, good news, and becoming a trusted confidante. Consider the "head, heart, and hands" approach as you continue to investigate this fascinating and challenging field.

Reflective Questions

For Those Individuals Considering Pursuing a Career in Nursing

- Why do you want to be a nurse?
- What particular aspects of nursing appeal to you?
- Have you had personal experiences that led to your interest in healthcare?
- Can you identify any career goals within the nursing profession?

- Have you ever followed/interacted with another health care professional you admire?
- Consider opportunities to shadow nurses, volunteer in a health care setting, or take a certified nursing assistant course to gain firsthand exposure to the nursing profession.

For Those Individuals Considering Returning to Academia

- As an LPN or RN returning to school to advance their nursing career, where do you think you "fit"?
- What do you consider advantages to your return?
- What do you consider challenges?

For Veteran Nurses

- What information would you share with a prospective student to help them understand what nurses do?
- What reasons do you have for being satisfied with choosing nursing as a career, considering challenges in the field right now?
- If you have mentored students during your career, what was the experience like for you?/for the student?

Food for Thought

Gratitude for Those Who Paved Our Way

My mother did not work outside the home. I doubt it was her first career choice. In the '50s and early '60s, it was rare in our sheltered world for mothers to work. When my mother was first married and later pregnant with my sister, she had to leave her job as secretary to the bank vice president. She loved that job, but the conventional "wisdom" of the day prevented her from working while pregnant.

My mother was not afforded a traditional bridal experience. There was no white wedding gown. She wore a wedding "suit" during their brief ceremony by the baptismal font. My parents could not enter the church beyond the vestibule, as she was Protestant and my father was Catholic. My mother had to promise that she would raise her children Catholic. Despite these sacrifices, she was a frequent worshipper at the local Methodist church, only a mile from our family's Catholic church.

Because housing after World War II was scarce, my parents and grandparents split the cost of a one family home. My mother and grandmother ruled the roost in the kitchen. We would set and clear the table, wash and dry the dishes, keep our rooms clean, and weed the hedges, but as daughters, we never learned to cook! It was too much chaos, they said; we would get "underfoot" in the small kitchen, they told us. Years later, my new husband was the unlucky beneficiary of my lack of culinary skills. I became a pretty decent cook minus a few untoward experiments.

During our time in elementary school, we were able to come home for lunch daily. There was always a meal waiting for us. Even though we lived close to the elementary school, I have no idea how we made it back and forth in the time allotted. I don't think we even had an hour to accomplish this feat. Knowing time was limited, my mother and grandmother were miracle workers, who made sure we were fed and on our way. They never missed a beat.

At one point, there were over ten people living in the five-bedroom home: my parents, siblings, grandparents, great-grandfather ("Big Grandpa"), our uncle, and his son. It never seemed crowded to us. We loved it. We never needed a babysitter, and there was always something going on or someone coming to visit. We usually had a roast for supper, probably because it was most cost-effective. Standard fare with the roasted meat always included peas and mashed potatoes on the nightly menu (it seemed that way to 6-year-old me, anyway). To this day, I cannot eat those two foods.

I believe my mother was on to my game of smushing the peas and potatoes under my dinner plate and then volunteering to clear the table. But she let it go, recognizing that it was easier to ignore my behavior than to deal with my father and his philosophy of "sit-at-the-table-until-your-plate-is-clean" school of parenting. Spilling milk was also a major faux pas and set my father off big time. The spiller was usually me, dumping the standard, massive 12-ounce glass of milk at everyone's place setting (milk is off my list today too). I'd still be sitting there at the table gagging at the sight of those peas, potatoes, and milk if not for her intervention. The point of all of this is to illustrate that my mother sacrificed, supported, and covered for all of us on countless occasions in our lives.

My mother walked with us everywhere to the many different stores and shops in our community. Everyone knew each other by first names. Almost daily, she brought us to the local library. We became the good students and the avid readers we are today because of my mother's influence.

In the winter, my mother took us ice skating and sledding at Roger Williams Park. I can still picture her standing there for hours at the top of "Suicide Hill" watching us plodding up and sledding down this behemoth of a mountain (it seemed so at the time) bending over to help four girls lace their ice skates at the pond below. I know she was freezing standing there in her skirt and boots (pants were not the norm for women then) while we called to her continuously to "watch me!" do the same stunt over and over. I never saw her roll her eyes or remember her complaining. Hours later, we trudged home, exhausted, but not without a stop at the Newport Creamery for hot chocolate. She was kind of a pushover, if truth be told.

It was the same deal with trips to the ocean. I think my mother and my father loved the water even more than we did. But we did let my mom get a swim or two in before screaming to her to rate our body surfing prowess. She patiently watched and waved. We brought her all kinds of objects taken from the ocean and showed her countless rocks that made up South Shore's stony beach. She did shy away from the questionable sea creatures we dragged back from the trek to and from "Magumbeeland" with our cousins, our father, and our wise-cracking uncle. Mom and my aunt made an effort to feign interest in our smelly treasures, which somehow mysteriously disappeared on the car ride home.

Over the years, my mother held steadfast to her role. My mother's unconditional regard and support for her children, husband, and family were truly remarkable and will always be remembered with gratitude and love. As in all families, there were hills and valleys in our childhood and adolescence. My mother helped us to weather those storms. I truly believe that her children are here in the positions we hold today because of her unwavering loyalty and belief in us.

References

Abu-Baker, N. N., AbuAlrub, S., Obeidat, R. F., & Assmairan, K. (2021). Evidence-based practice beliefs and implementations: A cross-sectional study among undergraduate nursing students. *BMC Nursing*, *20*(1), 1–8.

American Association of Colleges of Nursing. (2022, October). *Employment of new nurse graduates and employer preferences for baccalaureate-prepared nurses* (Research Brief 10-22). https://www.aacnnursing.org/Portals/0/PDFs/Data/Research-Brief-10-22.pdf

American Nurses Association. (2015). *Code of ethics for nurses with interpretive statements* (2nd ed.). https://www.nursingworld.org/practice-policy/nursing-excellence/ethics/code-of-ethics-for-nurses
American Nurses Association. (2021). *Nursing: Scope and standards of practice* (4th ed.).
Bell, S. G. (2020). Evidence-based practice competencies for RNs and APNs: How are we doing? *Neonatal Network, 39*(5), 299–302.
Carpenito, L. J. (2017). *Handbook of nursing diagnosis* (15th ed.). Wolters Kluwer.
Chichester, M. (2009). Passing the torch: Teaching the next generation of nurses. *Nursing for Women's Health,13(6)*, 507–510.
Culpepper, M., & Adams, P. (1988, July). Nursing in the Civil War. *American Journal of Nursing, 88*, 982.
Gordon, M. (1994). *Nursing diagnosis: Process and application* (3rd ed.). Mosby.
Harper, M. G., & Maloney, P. (Eds.). (2022). *Nursing professional development: Scope and standards of practice* (4th ed.). *Association for Nursing Professional Development.*
Hiriscau, E. I., Cauli, O., Donca, V., Marinescu, L. A., Macarie, A. E., Avram, L., Cancel, O. G., Donca, S., Buzdugan, E. C., Crisan, D. A., & Bodolea, C. (2024). The association between functional health patterns and frailty in hospitalized geriatric patients. *Geriatrics (Basel, Switzerland)*, *9*(2), 41. https://doi.org/10.3390/geriatrics90200
Karimi, H., & Masoudi Alavi, N. (2015). Florence Nightingale: The mother of nursing. *Nursing and Midwifery Studies, 4*(2), e29475. https://doi.org/10.17795/nmsjournal29475
Lotfi, M., Zamanzadeh, V., Khodayari-Zarnaq, R., & Mobasseri, K. (2021). Nursing process from theory to practice: Evidence from the implementation of "coming back to existence caring model" in burn wards. *Nursing Open*, *8*(5), 2794–2800. https://doi.org/10.1002/nop2.856
Mackey, A., & Bassendowski, S. (2017). The history of evidence-based practice in nursing education and practice. *Journal of Professional Nursing, 33*(1), 51–55.
McGrath, J. (2005). Critical thinking and evidence-based practice. *Journal of Professional Nursing*, *21*(6), 264–371.
National Council of State Boards of Nursing. (2024). *Active RN licenses.*
Picker Institute. (2013a). *Patient-centered care: The road ahead.* https://ipfcc.org/resources/Patient-Centered-Care-The-Road-Ahead.pdf
Picker Institute. (2013b). *Picker principles of patient centered care*. http://www.pickereurope.org/about-us/principles-of-patient-centred-care/
Saad, L. (2025, January 13). *Americans' ratings of U.S. professions stay historically low.* Gallup. https://news.gallup.com/poll/655106/americans-ratings-professions-stay historicallylow.aspx#:~:text=Honesty%20and%20ethical%20standards%20of%2023%20professions%2C%20rated%20in%20December,officers%2C%20pharmacists%20and%20medical%20doctors
Samios, G. (2025). *Prediction to practice.* Forbes Councils Member/Wolters Kluwer. https://www.forbes.com/councils/forbesbusinesscouncil/2025/02/18/from-prediction-to-practice-ais-role-in-healthcare-2025/
Shah, H. M., & Chung, K. C. (2009). Archie Cochrane and his vision for evidence-based medicine. *Plastic and Reconstructive Surgery*, *124*(3), 982–988. https://doi.org/10.1097/PRS.0b013e3181b03
Shaikh, U., & Lachman, P. (2021). Using the head, heart, and hands to manage change in clinical quality improvement in the time of COVID-19. *JQHC Communications,1*(1), 1–3. https://doi.org/10.1093/ijcoms/lyab012
Sipos, Y., Battisti, B., & Grimm, K. (2008). Achieving transformative sustainability learning: engaging head, hands and heart. *International Journal of Sustainability in Higher Education*, *9*(1), 68–86.
Smiley, R. A., Allgeyer, R. L., Shobo, Y., Lyons, K. C., Letourneau, R., Zhong, E., Kaminski Ozturk, N., & Alexander, M. (2023, April). The 2022 national nursing workforce survey. *Journal of Nursing Regulation*, *14*(1), Supplement 2, S1–S90.
Toney-Butler, T., & Thayer, J. (2023). *Nursing process.* StatPearls Publishing. https://www.ncbi.nlm.nih.gov/books/NBK499937/
U.S. Bureau of Labor Statistics. (2022). Occupational outlook handbook: Registered nurses.

Figure Credits

Fig. 1.1: Generated using Google Gemini.
Fig. 1.2: Stacey Richards, Nursing Documentation Principles, https://www.rch.org.au/rchcpg/hospital_clinical_guideline_index/nursing-documentation-principles/. Copyright © 2023 by The Royal Children's Hospital Melbourne.
Fig. 1.3: Marita G. Titler et al., "The Iowa Model of Evidence-Based Practice to Promote Quality Care," *Critical Care Nursing Clinics of North America*, vol. 13, no. 4, p. 500, https://www.sciencedirect.com/science/article/abs/pii/S0899588518300170. Copyright © 2001 by Elsevier B.V.

PART II

2 Critical Incidents

■ CHAPTER 2

The Critical Incident

Change

Progress is impossible without change, and those who cannot change their minds cannot change anything.

—George Bernard Shaw

Introduction

The following pages represent the voices of nurses in various roles and levels of practice. Beginning with Chapter 2, this next section of *Head, Heart, and Hands* addresses significant concepts within the nursing profession. These concepts are defined through the individual stories, or "critical incidents," that nurses have experienced in their work. Following each critical incident, nurse authors reflect on the decisions made, theorists and theories relevant to the event, factors playing into these decisions, and how the critical incident contributed to the way they view their professional practice.

Critical incidents are those experiences that challenge the skills, decision-making, and resilience of nurses (Alphonso, 2007). Critical incidents prompt nurses to reflect on their actions, feelings, and overall experiences, leading them to recognize significant insights and lessons learned. By examining what went well and what they might have done differently, nurses can identify areas for improvement and further refine their practice. Reflection fosters understanding of nurses' emotional responses, strengths, and limitations, fostering self-awareness, resilience, and coping skills with future professional challenges.

Critical incidents also promote the application of theory to practice by linking classroom learning to the intricacies of direct patient care. Examining critical incidents can bring to light those areas in health care settings needing improvement. This focused attention can lead to positive practice changes, increased patient safety, and staff role satisfaction, which promotes a culture of continuous learning and improvement (Fridlund et al., 2017).

Critical Incident One

The New Graduate

Change is a very complicated and intricate experience that is interrelated with nursing practice. Resistance to change in nursing can be expected, and as such is considered an important challenge in health care professions. Understanding the reasons for this resistance can help conquer this challenge in nursing (Cheraghi et al., 2023).

As a new grad, I participated in a few rapid responses and codes but always felt lost and not sure what to do. I used to think that being on my own and knowing when to call a rapid response...being an efficient member of it...would be a great unknown to me. To those who are not familiar—rapid responses/codes get very busy, with lots of staff in the room, many orders being given within seconds, organizing roles of the staff...all of this can be overwhelming. Having completed the new grad program, I was on my own,

At the beginning of the shift, I went to introduce myself to the first patient and bring her pm meds. She had been refusing meds all day and presented as anxious and angry. When I walked into the room, she let me know she did not want anything from the start. She did allow me to take her BP—which was low—and pt was tachycardic, in 120's. I contacted the provider, who came by the bedside to assess her and to encourage her to take her meds. As time went on, her condition worsened, systolic going to 70's, HR to 140's, agitated and screaming (pt was full code), necessitating rapid response. At that moment, my fears disappeared. I was able to compose myself, and work with the MD and team (me as a primary nurse) to calm pt down, administer meds, even give tasks to other members. I did not "freak out" but became the composed nurse I always admired in other nurses as they acted in these situation. The patient stabilized. I continued to observe her closely watching while caring for three other patients, but I was proud of myself: "Maybe I can do this?! Maybe I can be a good nurse." My confidence grew, and from that moment, instead of worrying, I was able to "dive into my job"—loving every bit of it. Do I still stress at times? Of course I do! And even after a year, in new situations, I sometimes feel like a novice. But it gets better every day, with every new skill I gain.

Relevant to this scenario is Dr. Patricia Benner's "Novice to Expert" theory, which comprises five levels of nursing experience. As described by Ozdemir (2019), Benner describes the levels: novice, a beginner with no experience; advanced beginner, who has gained some experience in actual nursing situations; competent, a nurse who has 1 to 2 years of experience in the same job field; proficient, a nurse who understands situations as whole parts; and expert, a nurse who no longer relies on principles, rules, or guidelines to connect to situations and determine actions.

In the previous situation, this graduate truly feels the experience of the novice nurse. Initially unsure of what to do, with a preceptor for guidance, she was able to step in and advocate for the patient. With time, experience and the mentoring support of role models, she clearly demonstrates positive progression through these experiential levels. After a year in practice (Ozdemir, 2019), she considers herself as "competent"; however, in some new situations, she admits to "still feeling like the novice."

Critical Incident Two

Why I Became a Nurse

My critical incident takes me back to a memorable Christmas Eve, many years ago. I had been working as a paramedic for approximately a year and had no aspirations to attend nursing school, nor change my career away from prehospital medicine. My partner and I were dispatched to a "cardiac arrest with bystander CPR in progress" at an address of a 42-year-old male we had come to know from bringing him to the emergency department for complications of the pancreatic cancer he had been diagnosed with 6 months prior. As my partner was the senior paramedic on scene and our truck could transport a patient, we were given report and took over care of the patient. My partner and I, along with two city paramedics, entered what many prehospital medical providers refer to as "the zone." While in "the zone" mindset, you ignore that you are working on a person, or that it is someone you know, or that you know their family. The situation becomes an extension of your training where nothing matters except what you should be doing in that moment for a patient in that situation. In a situation like this, emotions are shut off and shelved for later processing. The paramedics on that truck did everything they could, and on all accounts, we did it perfectly.

Unfortunately, the patient passed away at the hospital shortly, about 2 minutes after we delivered him to the emergency department physician. The physician would later write in an email to my company that more accurate and well-performed care could not have been accomplished by a team of experienced physicians. However well we had done our jobs, I was devastated. I sat on the tailgate of my ambulance, and I cried. I cried because we did everything for this young man, and he still died. The responding team treated this patient accurately, in a timely manner, and with precision, yet I was devastated that I could not do more for this patient. I cried because my best made no difference for this patient.

My senior partner came out to the truck, handed me a bottle of cold Diet Coke from the hospital vending machine and made a statement to me that I remember even today. My partner said, "You must think an awful lot of yourself to think you can cheat death, kid. You showed up, used all your skills as best you could, and did a job that few can. You even did it better than most. The patient still died. He was lucky. Hopefully, someone with your skills will show up and do their best for you. Then you'll be lucky too. But what's more is you care. You care for that patient and his family. You honestly care that you couldn't do more. You feel like you let that patient down. You're no paramedic at heart, kid. Go be more. Go to nursing school or something." While I do not agree that I am not a paramedic at heart or in the sentiment that paramedics do not care about their patients, I did start applying to nursing schools that next spring. I still see my partner from that day often as he is a paramedic whose company services the area my hospital is in. He still quips "See? I told you that you care. I'm glad I told you to be more."

This nurse describes a former career in emergency medicine filled with many critical incidents. His time as a paramedic still influences his nursing career even today and aligns with a key component of the teachings of a prominent nursing theorist, Jean Watson, and her Theory of Transpersonal Caring (Watson, 2008).

Watson's theory and her use of ten "carative" factors differentiate nurses from other health care providers and highlights what is special about us. No other health care providers are lauded for their empathy, caring, and ability to advocate for a patient and their family. Jean Watson's theory organizes these characteristics and presents them as our strength.

Watson's tenet of being authentically present and healing through kindness are pearls that I repeat to myself in my daily work even in a supervisory role. I have said to many new nurses, "I can teach you what drugs to put in a syringe, but I can't teach you to care about grandma." I realize how glib that statement sounds; however, I believe that is true. You cannot teach a nurse to care, but if it is in their heart you can turn them into a wonderful nurse. Caring and empathy have always been so integral to my practice that I believe that is what my paramedic partner meant to say: that the amount of empathy and caring I always exhibited was more akin to a nurse than a paramedic. So that is what I have taken it in my heart to mean.

Change Theory: Kurt Lewin

Regarded as one of the modern pioneers of social, organizational, and applied psychology in the United States, **Kurt Lewin developed change theory** (Burnes, 2020). His model represents a dynamic balance of forces working in opposing directions and includes three key concepts: (1) driving forces, (2) restraining forces, and (3) equilibrium. These driving forces create a *push-pull* effect as an individual navigates through the process of change.

Restraining forces are those life experiences that oppose change (fears, threats), while driving forces inspire change (personal goals, career advancement). While driving forces steer individuals in a desired direction, causing a shift in the equilibrium toward change, restraining forces hinder change by sending individuals in the opposite direction. Equilibrium is a state of being where driving forces equal restraining forces. It is a condition where no change occurs but can be raised or lowered by changes occurring between the driving and restraining forces (Shirey, 2013; Wojciechowski et al., 2016).

Unfreezing, Change, and Refreezing

Lewin's most influential theory was his model of the change process in human systems. He theorized a three-stage model of change that is known as the *unfreezing-change-refreeze* model that rejects and replaces prior learning. This method involves preparing individuals for change, making those changes, and, finally, integrating and normalizing those changes within the organization (Wojciechowski et al., 2016).

Unfreezing involves the tendency of individuals to seek out an environment of relative safety to maintain a sense of control. Attaching their sense of identity to their environment creates stability for individuals from which any alternatives, even those that may offer significant benefit, will cause discomfort. Talking about the future will not necessarily transfer individuals from a *frozen* state. Substantial effort may be needed to *unfreeze* and motivate individuals for readiness to change. Some individuals are *change ready,* while others may need more to leave their comfort zones (Shirey, 2013).

Change focuses on the belief that change is a journey rather than a simple step. Change is difficult and requires considerable time and support. A typical barrier occurs when leaders spend time with their own personal journey, assuming that others should automatically follow suit. For many, the hardest part of this stage is in beginning the change. Individuals can become caught in situations where they are not accountable for the risks of work in transitioning and where talking about change is substituted for action (Shirey, 2013).

Refreezing entails putting down roots again and establishing a new place of stability. This stage is often rather tentative and can lead to a state of *slush*, where freezing is never attained. *Change shock* occurs in individuals working at low levels of productivity while waiting for the next change (Shirey, 2013).

Reflective Questions

As you answer the self-reflection questions below, consider the following suggestions:

Ask more "what" questions. When reflect on areas you want to change, "what" questions help you to be objective, helping you to focus and look forward to the future. This positive form of thinking can help you discover what has worked for you in the past.

Document your thoughts. Keep a journal and write frequently, even if your reflections are short. Making lists or creating sketches complement your words. Journal writing also shows concrete evidence of your progress over time.

Act on change. You may need to move on or let go of someone or something, whether it is an old behavior, limiting belief, pattern or a part of your identity or values system that no longer serves you.

Use past experiences with change. Given time and distance, this action provides the perspective to see change without judgment, for what it was rather than for how you wished it had been. Every time you review it broadens your view and provides you with wisdom for the present situation.

1. Are you in the middle of a transition (job change, living situation, long-term relationship)?
2. If you decide to keep your current habits, do you think your life be better or worse in a year?
3. What advice would you give your "future self" today?
4. What part of your life needs to change, and why haven't you done it yet?
5. What action can you take today that would make you proud?

Scenario

Role Transition

A graduate of an LPN-to-BSN program 6 months ago, who has completed hospital wide and unit orientation, Marcus works 32 hours weekly (evenings) on a 20-bed adult surgical unit. He was previously employed on this same unit as an LPN for over 5 years. Upon receiving his assignment tonight, Marcus learns that he will be responsible ("charge") for 12 patients on the unit. His team consists of an LPN, an RN, two certified nurse's aides (CNA), and a unit clerk. Marcus receives a report on the 12 patients:

- Five new postoperative clients; one is experiencing nausea and vomiting
- Two patients scheduled for surgery within the hour
- Four elderly patients requiring assistance with activities of daily living
- One patient, postoperative day two, at high risk for falls

The nursing supervisor calls to say that she is in the process of securing "extra help" for the unit tonight, expressing confidence in his abilities and his prior experience as an LPN.

In planning and delegation of this assignment, answer the following questions:

1. What questions does he have of his nursing supervisor?
2. What does Marcus need to know about his team members?
3. How does Marcus organize and prioritize the care of these clients?
4. What should the assignment sheet look like?

Food for Thought

Change Your Attitude: The Value of a Sense of Humor

Humor is the great thing, the saving thing after all.
The minute it crops up, all our hardnesses yield, all our irritations,
and resentments flit away, and a sunny spirit takes their place.

—Mark Twain

For nurses, possessing a sense of humor can ultimately lead to better self-esteem and self-competency. In the middle of a stressful time, humor serves as a pause to lessen the anxiety response; it helps to focus on what needs to be done. This is because humor and laughter stimulate the anterior cingulate cortex, an area of the brain associated with attention and decision-making (Lavin et al, 2013).

Standards of appropriateness, timing, and sensitivity are crucial elements in using humor respectfully with patients. To balance lightheartedness and professionalism, it is crucial to use humor in such a way as to prevent it from becoming a distraction. Humor in nursing can be a valuable tool to break the ice, foster rapport, and reduce stress for nurses, students, patients, and families. Applying humor thoughtfully has been shown to enhance the nurse-patient relationship (El-Sayed et al., 2024).

In caring for patients with medical challenges, "therapeutic humor" can sometimes do as much as the treatment (El-Sayed et al., 2024). Along with enhancing the immune system and reducing pain perception, humor can improve digestion and promote better sleep. Humor employed as a coping mechanism assists patients to "reframe" their illnesses and become better able to seek out support services.

Humor in the health care setting is not a continuous stream of quips and banter. Humor in patient care must be complemented by principles of nursing: empathy and compassion; acceptance and respect; and sincere, authentic communication. Winona Ball, RN, of Governors State University in Illinois stresses the importance of active listening on the part of nurses, which leads patients to "guide the humor" (Ball, n.d.)

Education in the benefits of humor across the life spectrum often finds its inception in families. Storytelling is an art form as well. Reliving family stories at reunions and annual get-togethers reduces them to tears, no matter how long ago the event happened.

Growing up, I used to think that it was normal for everyone's father to hang their head out the car window while driving, yelling comments at other drivers or passersby. Today, those actions would not produce the same results. If my dad was at the wheel when we had friends in the car, he would curb his language as he shouted at "bad" drivers. His favorite "outburst" was "Cock-a-doodle-doo!" when he thought the driver he passed was going too slowly, kept their blinker on, or showed any other number of what he felt were driving weaknesses.

In my dad's family, there were seven children, three boys and four girls; he was the second eldest. With such a big family, there was always a celebration. It didn't matter if it was a wedding or funeral. Even at my parents' 80th birthday party at a local clambake club, every event included the obligatory singing of "Bill Bailey" and "Danny Boy," recanting of stories from decades ago, taunting, joking, and laughter. Each person got a chance to come up to the microphone. You never knew what to expect: a song, a funny story, an off-color joke, or a "roast" of some relative. But what I remember best was the happiness of a family that, despite going through some tough times over the years, loved each other and celebrated each moment.

References

Alphonso, C. (2007). Reflection on a critical incident. *Contemporary Nurse*, *24*(1), 89–92. https://doi.org/10.5172/conu.2007.24.1.89

Ball, W. S. (n.d.). *Humor in nursing.* Nurse Plus Academy. Retrieved July 12, 2025, from https://nurse.plus/become-a-nurse/humor-in-nursing/

Burnes, B. (2020). The origins of Lewin's three-step model of change. *Journal of Applied Behavioral Science, 56*(1), 32–59. https://doi.org/10.1177/0021886319892685

Cheraghi, R., Ebrahimi, H., Kheibar, N., & Sahebihagh, M. H. (2023). Reasons for resistance to change in nursing: An integrative review. *BMC Nursing*, *22*(1), 310. https://doi.org/10.1186/s12912-023-01460-0

El-Sayed, M. M., AbdElhay, E. S., Hawash, M. M., & Mohamed Tah, S. (2024). The power of laughter: a study on humor and creativity in undergraduate nursing education in Egypt. *BMC Nursing, 23*(259). https://doi.org/10.1186/s12912-024-01913-0

Fridlund, B., Henricson, M., & Mårtensson, J. (2017). Critical incident technique applied in nursing and healthcare sciences. *SOJ Nursing & Health Care, 3*(1), 1–5. http://dx.doi.org/10.15226/2471-6529/3/1/00125

Lavin, C., Melis, C., Mikulan, E., Gelormini, C., Huepe, D., & Ibañez, A. (2013) The anterior cingulate cortex: an integrative hub for human socially-driven interactions. *Frontiers in Neuroscience*, *8*(7), 64. https://doi.org/10.3389/fnins.2013.00064

Ozdemir, N. G. (2019). The development of nurses' individualized care perceptions and practices: Benner's novice to expert model perspective.*International Journal of Caring Sciences, 12*(2), 1279–1285.

Shirey, M. R. (2013). Lewin's theory of planned change as a strategic resource. *The Journal of Nursing Administration*, *43*(2), 69–72. https://doi.org/10.1097/NNA.0b013e31827f20a9

Watson, J. (2008). *Nursing: The philosophy and science of caring.* University Press of Colorado.

Wojciechowski, E., Pearsall, T., Murphy, P., & French, E. (2016). A case review: Integrating Lewin's theory with lean's system approach for change. *Online Journal of Issues in Nursing,21*(2), 4. https://doi.org/10.3912/OJIN.Vol21No02Man04

CHAPTER 3

Caring

Never believe that a few caring people cannot change the world. For, indeed, that is all who ever have.

—Margaret Mead

Introduction

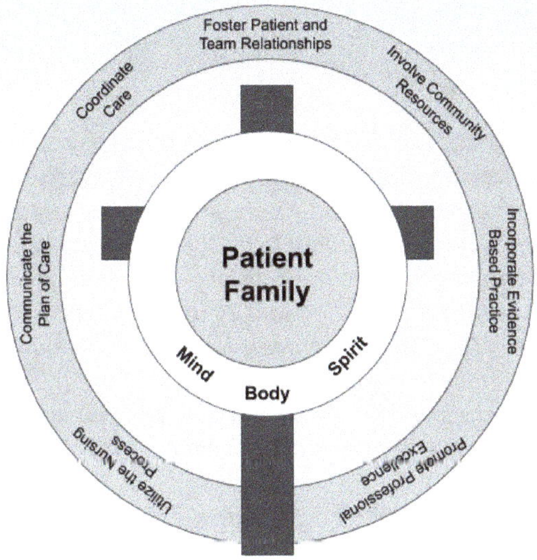

Figure 3.1 Watson's Theory of Caring
Created by Brian Duphily

Conceived as the "essence of the profession" by nurse theorist Jean Watson (2008), caring in nursing ranges far beyond carrying out physical tasks. Caring embodies empathy and compassion, promotes development of a therapeutic relationship, and builds trust between patient and caregiver. Caring's holistic approach encompasses physical, emotional, psychological, and spiritual needs. Patients feel respected, supported, and motivated in an environment that encourages participation and cultivates compliance with the plan of care. Additionally, the benefits of caring extend to providers. For nurses, compassionate caregiving has been shown to increase job satisfaction, emotional resilience, and personal growth (Molina-Mula & Gallo-Estrada, 2020).

In nursing, caring exemplifies a humanistic approach that links professional knowledge, clinical expertise, and moral values (Wong, 2025). Caring cultivates nurturing relationships for nurses and patients, creates an environment conducive to healing, and promotes holistic well-being. In her seminal work, Watson (2008) emphasizes that caring is so much more than a chore to be finished; it is an "essential way of being."

The two critical incidents included in this chapter are striking examples of caring. They clearly illustrate the importance of integrating the following key elements into nursing practice:

- **Active listening,** which conveys empathy and generates an atmosphere conducive to clearly understanding the information communicated between nurse and patient. This open, respectful interaction creates trust and empowers patients to feel heard and valued.
- **Empathy,** which involves understanding patients' feelings, experiences, and fears, in responding with genuine compassion. Empathetic care lessens anxiety, creates a sense of calm, and contributes to a positive patient experience.
- **Holism,** which is vital to understanding the essence of nursing. With this comprehensive approach to patient care, the nurse recognizes physical, mental, emotional, and spiritual well-being. By individualizing, identifying, and prioritizing health care needs, this approach supports timely, collaborative, and comprehensive intervention in the patient's overall health and recovery.

Critical Incident One

The Art of Listening

In my first and most trying year, I met MS while working on a busy cardiac telemetry unit, with a nursing ratio of 1:6 on the evening shift. At change of shift, I received report and discharge papers on MS, an older gentleman with chest pain (CP). He was a typical CP rule out, (labs/imaging normal, no chest pain). I entered a crowded room to discharge MS. While reviewing discharge information, MS described gastrointestinal pain. His family also mentioned that his usual voracious appetite had decreased significantly, leading to a 20 lb weight loss in the last 6 months. I noted too that Mr. Smith had eaten 5%–10% of his meals in the past 24 hours. MS remarked that "food doesn't seem to sit right." I spoke to the discharging doctor about my concerns regarding MS, his decreased appetite and weight loss over an extended period that was not the norm for him. This doctor took my concerns seriously, canceled the discharge, and ordered abdominal imaging for him.

MS had advanced colon cancer. I discharged him the next evening after a hematology/oncology consult with an outpatient appointment. Unfortunately, the prognosis was not good. Several months later while at work, one of MS's daughters came to invite me to his funeral. She stated nothing could have changed the outcome, but the care her father received allowed him to prepare for his death. He was able to get his affairs in order, spend time with his family, and reconnect with Army buddies he had not seen in decades.

This event highlighted how essential it is for nurses to LISTEN to their patients. That night, I was terribly busy, scared of making a mistake, and wanted to be as fast as the other nurses. It would have been easy for me to fall into a task-oriented tunnel vision. However, something made me hear him. Meeting MS made a significant difference in how I have practiced nursing through the years, that is, to make a concerted effort to not only hear my patients, but to listen.

Hildegard E. Peplau's Interpersonal Relation Theory aptly applies here (Hagerty et al., 2017). Peplau emphasizes how the relationship between nurse and patient can encourage forward progression for both individuals. Peplau theorized that nurse-patient relationships must have characteristics of respect, empathy, and active listening throughout the three main phases of nurse/patient interaction (orientation, working, and termination) to be successful (Hagerty et al., 2017). Peplau's interpersonal relation theory serves to highlight the factors at play during the interaction with patient MS and serves as a daily guide in this nurse's effective and therapeutic communication skills in her professional practice.

Critical Incident Two

The Depth of Human Connection That Nursing Demands

During my first month as a new ADN graduate working in the emergency department, I encountered a critical incident that significantly shaped my perspective on nursing. A middle-aged patient arrived via ambulance in cardiac arrest. Despite our team's swift efforts—initiating CPR, administering medications, and defibrillating—the patient did not survive. When the code was called, the room fell silent, leaving an overwhelming emotional weight.

Before transitioning to nursing, I worked as a paramedic for several years. During that time, I handled many cardiac arrests, often arriving at scenes, performing resuscitative efforts, and transporting patients to the emergency department. While those experiences exposed me to high-stakes situations, my role as a paramedic typically ended once the patient was handed off. Rarely did I witness the human aftermath—the raw grief of families or the emotional resonance of loss.

What made this incident critical was not only the gravity or nature of the situation but also the interactions that followed. As a nurse, I found myself sitting with the grieving family after they were given the devastating news. Their pain was palpable, and for the first time, I truly understood the depth of human connection that nursing demands. Offering words of comfort and simply being present in their sorrow underscores the importance of empathy and communication in this profession. The aftermath of the incident was multifaceted. Personally, I grappled with feelings of sadness, placing myself in the surviving family members' shoes. Professionally, it reinforced the importance of teamwork, emotional resilience, and reflection. I sought support from colleagues and participated in a debriefing session, which helped me process the event and learn from it. Moving forward, I became more proactive in self-care and in seeking mentorship to navigate the emotional challenges of emergency nursing.

This incident profoundly influenced my professional practice. It highlighted the dual role of a nurse as both a clinical expert and a compassionate caregiver. I am learning to balance these roles and prioritize effective communication with patients and their families, even in the most difficult moments. In contrast to my paramedic role, which prioritized clinical tasks, I've come to appreciate the holistic nature of nursing—attending not only to physical needs but also to emotional and spiritual well-being. Reflecting on my past as a paramedic, I've learned to bridge the gap between clinical expertise and human connection. Nursing extends far beyond the technicalities of saving lives.

Jean Watson's theory of human caring (Watson, 2008) emphasizes the holistic nature of nursing, focusing on caring (including self-care) as the essence of the profession. Watson identifies ten carative factors (Caritas Processes), which include cultivating sensitivity to oneself and others, developing a helping-trusting relationship, and providing a supportive environment. Her theory advocates addressing not just the physical needs of patients but also their emotional, social, and spiritual well-being.

This theory aligns closely with the experience of sudden death. Watson's emphasis on creating a caring-healing environment resonated with the approach to comforting the grieving family. While the technical aspects of care (e.g., CPR and advanced life support) were vital during the code, it was the human connection and empathy that made a lasting impact afterward. The nurse becomes a leading character in a story that people will relive over and over again. Watson's theory guides ongoing practice. It reminds us to approach every patient and family interaction with intentionality and compassion, recognizing that these moments—even in crisis—are opportunities for healing beyond the physical.

Reflective Questions

After reading this chapter

1. What role do you feel caring plays in the nursing profession?
2. What concepts play a major role in caring?
3. How does caring build trust between nurse and patient?
4. What do you feel is the impact of caring on patient outcomes?

Scenario

Applying "The Essence of Nursing" to Practice

Employed in the emergency department (ED) at a local 400 bed hospital for 15 years, Alyssa (RN) recognizes that during her shift, there is an unusually heavy caseload. Working with Alyssa at this time are two other licensed individuals: Martha (RN, 5 years) and Raymond (LPN, 6 years).

A 40-year-old male presents to the ED with symptoms of dehydration and heat stroke. He shows signs of altered consciousness, a rapid heartbeat, and low blood pressure. Following an initial assessment by Alyssa, the task of starting the patient on a 0.9% normal saline IV has fallen to Raymond, who began administering intravenous therapy approximately three weeks ago, following successful completion of a hospital-wide, state nursing board approved IV therapy course. Alyssa delegates the intravenous drip procedure to Ray to assist the ED nurse manager (MSN) with a trauma patient who just arrived in the ED.

Although Alyssa has not personally supervised Raymond during IV administration, she knows that he demonstrates competence in other nursing tasks. When Martha offers to administer the IV, Raymond states he is comfortable with the task. Martha states that she will "check back soon," and if any problems should arise, she is to be notified immediately.

Questions

1. What is the general scope of practice for nurses governing the task of administering IV saline? Are there exceptions to these requirements?
2. Given the condition of the patient (dehydration and heat stroke) and Raymond's experience with administering IV fluids, what might be the potential consequences of improperly placed IV line, or failure to access a vein for this patient?
3. Because supervision was unavailable at the time, how might the nurses in this scenario collaborate to reconsider the delegation of tasks to achieve safe outcomes for this patient?

Food for Thought

Applying Holistic Care in Reading With Patients

> *It is not enough to simply teach children to read; we have to give them something worth reading. Something that will stretch their imaginations to help them make sense of their own lives and encourage them to reach out toward people whose lives are quite different from their own.*
>
> *—Katherine Patterson*

As mentioned earlier in this chapter, meeting individuals' care needs "encompasses physical, emotional, psychological, and spiritual" elements (Watson, 2008). In nursing, these needs can be met through a number of creative ways and may include many different patient populations and scenarios across the life span. I understand that the following content may seem unconventional to some, and warrants some explanation, so please bear with me.

Growing up in the city, we spent many hours at the library, conveniently located nearby our home. My family and I are avid readers today because of this experience. We have noticed, too, that we gravitate to others who have similarly cultivated a love of reading. There is not a discussion with friends and family that does not include a book being mentioned and/or debated.

So it was not unusual for me to blend this passion as part of the "caring connection" in my nursing career, working among the many diverse settings with the populations I encountered—namely, patients, students, and colleagues. Throughout my nursing career, I have been able to integrate Watson's caring's theory, and its related holistic approach, to the books I have shared with patients: working 11–7 in the pediatric unit, rocking a sick child; sitting by a scared 4-year-old's bedside in the middle of the night when he was missing his mom and dad; or sharing and discussing books with residents of nursing homes during the nurse-patient daily routine.

As a community health nurse working for the Visiting Nurse Association (VNA) in Maternal Child Health (MCH), I shared books, ideas, and questions on varied subjects with the patients and their families who welcomed me into their homes. This seemingly insignificant component of care sparked awareness and discussion of topics such as parenting, nutrition, and growth and developmental milestones. More importantly, it highlighted the benefits of reading.

In conducting a service-learning initiative in our community college's nursing program, we created a weekly "Parents Group" in the city's local library. The staff there graciously opened their Children's Room to us weekly to conduct these educational sessions. Supervised by nursing faculty, nursing students developed a weekly age-appropriate activity, along with a nutritious snack, followed by reading stories to the children. In an adjoining room, moms and dads were free to discuss their current parenting questions, establish informal support groups, make lifelong friends, and share parenting books, resources, and tips. The program was well received and well attended. These grassroots efforts can effectively drive change and raise awareness.

Over the many semesters of teaching, together with students, we developed a summer reading list each year (not textbooks!) of the many books whose titles and content emerged in both class discussions and clinical post conferences. Each year, both students and teachers anticipated receiving that inventory of "not required" summer reading. "Put that on the list!" was a frequent request if a book idea surfaced during class.

And finally, I have many fond memories of reading to both my children and the pediatric patients I had the good fortune to meet. I couldn't decide on just one story, so here are my top four:

The Monster at the End of This Book by Jon Stone

Based on their hilarious reactions every time we read this story together, I would place this book at the top of the list. Children came to know the story by heart. The main character, *Sesame Street's* lovable, furry Grover, is horrified to learn that there is a monster at the end of the book and begs the reader not to finish it, to avoid the monster. He uses several methods to keep us away, such as cementing them together with bricks. Mimicking Grover, my kids would shout, "Don't turn the page! Don't you know there's a monster at the end of this book?!" No matter how hard Grover tried to keep his readers from turning the pages, he could not prevent them from discovering who the monster actually is. What makes the book so funny is the twist at the end: The "monster" is Grover himself. "I am so embarrassed!" the kids would shriek, along with Grover. It was a very noisy reading experience.

Blueberries for Sal by Robert McCloskey

This classic tale of two mothers, two children, and a bucket of blueberries brings back memories of picking low-bush blueberries in summer. Affectionately known as "The Blueberries Book," Little Sal goes out blueberry picking with her mother on Blueberry Hill. Her mother's plan was to pick enough blueberries to can for the winter. Sal's plan was to stuff herself on blueberries. Kids love the description of the blueberries hitting the bottom of the pail: "Kuplink, Kuplank, Kuplunk." While Sal and her mother were picking berries on one side of the hill, Mama Bear and Little Bear were on the other side with the same plan. While Sal's mother and Mama Bear were collecting berries, Sal and Little Bear wander away to rest. Somehow, the two switch places and come face-to-face with the wrong mother. After a moment of confusion, it all works out. Little Sal and Little Bear reunite with their mothers and hurry down Blueberry Hill for home.

Where the Wild Things Are by Maurice Sendak

Many lessons here for new parents! This was a well-worn favorite. We can all relate to bedtime protests, as well as the concept of time-out. In this story, after his mother sends him to bed without dinner, Max falls asleep. His room transforms into a forest surrounded by ocean, with a boat waiting for him. Excited for the chance to travel to a faraway land and escape his mother's rules, Max lands in a place where the "wild things" live: huge, ferocious but actually tame creatures. They try to scare Max off by roaring and baring their teeth and claws. The wild things soon recognize that Max is the wildest of all of them and make him their king. After a "rumpus" of dancing, stomping, and swinging through the trees, Max has had enough. He starts to miss his mother, leaves the wild things and sails back home. He smells the food that he wasn't allowed to eat waiting for him in his bedroom: "And it is still hot." Max is allowed to express his feelings with the wild rumpus, returning home when he's worked it all out (a time-out in his bedroom). I love this book for all its lessons. It teaches us about emotions, imagination, and limit-setting with love and helps us recognize the value of regrouping through creative channeling of feelings.

Goodnight Moon by Margaret Wise Brown

This story emphasizes the importance of rituals. As I read this book to children, I always wondered if the routine, short of asking for yet another glass of water or to check the closet for monsters, was the bunny's way of delaying bedtime. He could not rest until he bid goodnight to each and every item in the room: a red balloon, a pair of socks, a dollhouse, a bowl of mush, and two kittens. As the story continues, the bunny gets more and more tired before finally saying "Goodnight noises everywhere," just as he falls asleep. My own kids loved to embellish these items ("stinky" socks, "rotting" mush), laughing themselves silly with their own descriptive contributions. I am positive this was their ploy to delay bedtime.

References

Hagerty, T. A., Samuels, W., Norcini-Pala, A., & Gigliotti, E. (2017). Peplau's theory of interpersonal relations: An alternate factor structure for patient experience data. *Nursing Science Quarterly, 30*(2), 160–167. https://doi.org/10.1177/0894318417693286

Molina-Mula, J., & Gallo-Estrada, J. (2020). Impact of nurse-patient relationship on quality of care and patient autonomy in decision-making. *International Journal of Environmental Research and Public Health*, *17*(3), 835. https://doi.org/10.3390/ijerph17030835

Watson, J. (2008). *Nursing: The philosophy and science of caring.* University Press of Colorado.

Wong, F. M. F. (2025). Fostering caring attributes to improve patient care in nursing through small-group work: Perspectives of students and educators. *Nursing Reports*, *15*(1), 10. https://doi.org/10.3390/nursrep15010010

Figure Credit

Fig. 3.1: Generated using Google Gemini.

■ CHAPTER 4

Integrating Theory and Evidence-Based Practice

Nurses are not just doers. Our work is supported by evidence and guided by theory. We integrate evidence and theory with our knowledge of patients and make important decisions with and for patients and families at the point of care. Research and practice are not separate but integrated. Nursing is a practice discipline with our own theories and research base that we both generate, use, and disseminate to others.

—Antonia Villarruel, Dean of Nursing, University of Pennsylvania School of Nursing

Introduction

Evidence-based practice (EBP) integrates current research data with clinical expertise and patient values to inform decision-making. Nursing interventions based on scientific evidence lead to improved patient outcomes through the provision of current, best practices. Merging nursing theories with EBP reinforces a patient-centered approach through the provision of sound care, incorporating individual preferences, values, and cultures. This connection closes the gap between research and patient-centered care and reinforces the effect of nurses' evidence-based interventions (Baptiste, 2023; Ominyi & Alabi, 2025).

Nursing theories unravel the intricacies of patient care by providing physiological, psychological, and sociocultural aspects of health and illness. When coupled with EBP, these theories guide clinical decision-making by supporting interventions with theory-based foundations for practice. As an example, Baptiste (2023) cites Watson's "theory of human caring," which emphasizes the importance of establishing a caring and empathetic nurse-patient relationship. By integrating this theory into EBP, nurses are encouraged to prioritize patient communication and emotional support, leading to a more holistic and patient-centered care approach.

Beneficial to nursing practice, the incorporation of nursing theory into EBP encourages critical appraisal of research literature. When nurses are well versed in theoretical concepts, they can evaluate research studies with a deeper understanding of the underlying principles. This empowers nurses to connect and apply research findings to specific patient scenarios.

Additionally, incorporating nursing theories into practice helps nurses to recognize the patient as an individual. Each patient has separate and distinct preferences, values, and cultural needs. A personalized, holistic approach can foster collaboration in planning care and ultimately lead to positive outcomes for both patient and nurse (Ominyi & Alabi, 2025).

Merging research and patient-centered care provides nurses with a comprehensive approach in their assessments, tailoring interventions to recognize patients' unique, individual needs. This coupling balances theoretical knowledge with empirical precision and consistency, leading to care that is informed, current, holistic, patient-centered, and ethically grounded.

Nurturing this collaboration is vital to furthering the profession as well as protecting the patients in our care.

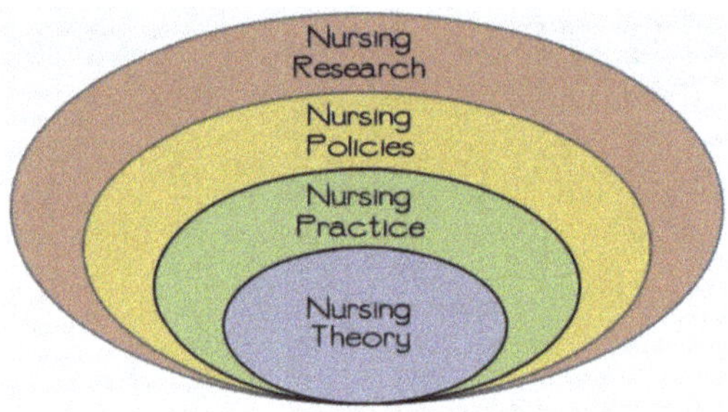

Figure 4.1 Interrelationship Between Nursing Theory, Practice, Policies, and Research

The two critical incidents introduced in Chapter 4 illustrate the importance of the connection between nursing theory and real-world decision-making. Readers are introduced to evidence-based care and collaboration through Imogene King's theory of goal attainment, as well as the grief theory of Elizabeth Kübler-Ross. The integration of theory and practice is noted with the nurses' discussion of utilizing both practice "skills" to make decisions and navigate through the psychosocial issues surfacing in their respective experiences.

Knowledge of the stages of grief, coupled with the value of empathy, exemplify those characteristics, skills, and tools that a nurse must possess to support patients. The nurses in these two critical incidents recognize and address the fact that each patient is unique; therefore, the plan should include individualizing the care to the patient in every situation.

The insights expressed by the writers here illustrate the danger when nurses' feelings are "put aside" during critical incidents. These feelings build and can lead to compassion fatigue and burnout. The importance of "debriefing" following traumatic, tragic events is an important life lesson that can improve one's personal growth as a nurse. This growth can be measured when revisiting past situations and reflecting how the approach might have been different, or in validating that growth occurred.

Critical Incident One

Theory to Practice: Guiding Patients Through Loss and Grief

Learn to get in touch with the silence within yourself and know that everything in life has purpose. There are no mistakes, no coincidences, all events are blessings given to us to learn.

—Elisabeth Kübler-Ross

I cared for a patient who succumbed to stage 4 cancer, leaving behind young children. The emotional gravity of the situation was profound, especially as I witnessed the family grappling with their loss. The children's confusion and pain were heartbreaking, and their mother's passing left a palpable void in the room. The event was "critical" because it underscores the complexity of nursing care during end-of-life moments. This situation required both clinical knowledge and profound emotional resilience to support the family. The death of a parent with young children is particularly devastating, as it disrupts the family dynamic and leaves lingering emotional scars. In the immediate aftermath, I prioritized comforting the family, offering emotional support, and ensuring they understood the available resources. The health care team arranged grief counseling and connected the family with social services for additional support. The patient's passing served as a somber reminder of the inevitability of death, even with the best care. For the fam-

ily, the loss marked the beginning of a long grieving process. Despite their pain, they expressed gratitude for the compassionate care provided. Professionally, this experience reaffirmed the necessity of self-care and peer support to process such emotionally heavy incidents. This incident emphasized the significance of presence and empathy in nursing practice. It deepened my understanding of the human connection that defines nursing.

This experience shaped the attending nurse's approach to end-of-life care. It highlights the need to integrate palliative principles and foster a supportive environment for patients and their families. Elisabeth Kübler-Ross's five stages of grief theory (Kübler-Ross, 1969) provides a framework for understanding the emotional responses individuals experience during significant loss. The stages include denial, anger, bargaining, depression, and acceptance. These stages are not linear but offer insight into the grieving process and how individuals cope with profound emotional pain. Kübler-Ross's work emphasizes the importance of empathy, active listening, and support during grief, which is integral to nursing care, especially in end-of-life scenarios (Kübler-Ross, 1969).

By understanding where individuals might be within these stages, nurses can effectively tailor an individualized approach to meet their emotional needs and those of the grieving family members. For example, during the critical incident, the nurse here noted that the family fluctuated between denial and depression stages. Using this framework afforded the nurse the opportunity to offer the support appropriate for these stages.

Kübler-Ross's theory is directly applicable to the critical incident described. The stages of grief provide a lens by which the nurse can attempt to understand and address the family's emotional state. Recognizing the family's initial denial helped this nurse to intervene appropriately, and to effectively communicate, clearly and compassionately. This incident highlighted the value of informed practice, represented by this nurse's application of the five stages of grief in guiding nursing interventions and ensuring holistic care for patients and their loved ones (Kübler-Ross & Kessler, 2005).

Critical Incident Two

Evidence-Based Collaborative Care in the Home Health Setting

I work in the home health setting, caring for a 25-year-old male client diagnosed with Duchenne muscular dystrophy, since his discharge from the hospital, where he had a gastrostomy PEG tube placed, a tracheostomy, and now requires 24/7 ventilator dependence. This was my first job working as a nurse. I did not feel fully trained for the severity of the patient. I learned a lot from the team of specialists involved in his home care: The respiratory therapist guided me in ventilator operation, settings, and troubleshooting problems; the physical therapist reviewed the Hoyer lift in transfers from bed to mechanical chair; and the wound specialist offered tips in caring for the stoma site for the gastrostomy tube. This experience demonstrated the importance of collaboration with the health care team and continual education to properly assess for change of condition and apply evidenced-based nursing interventions. I am learning how to work with specialists, evaluate medication effectiveness based on condition changes, and, most importantly, to navigate essentially being a guest in another person's home. It can be difficult learning how to efficiently provide nursing services while respecting the boundaries and wishes of the client and family. I have established a positive rapport with the client and family, so I am able to be empathetic but direct regarding his plan of care. However, home care nurses cannot force our clients to do anything they do not want to do. Clients and families need to be a part of the decision-mak-

ing process regarding their care. They have a right to refuse. Our job is to continue educating and working with clients and families to ensure the best overall outcomes.

The nurse in this setting is a proponent of maintaining an evidence-based collaborative practice. A collaborative approach emphasizes the importance of partnership and shared decision-making, involving the nurse, patient, family, and other contributing health care professionals, where everyone actively participates in the patient's plan of care.

Imogene King's "theory of goal attainment" (Heron, 2023) describes the importance of initiating therapeutic nurse-patient communication early on in the relationship. In this critical incident, the home care nurse recognizes the importance of enhancing the plan with including the experience and expertise of physical, respiratory, and wound care therapists in collaborative goal setting to achieve optimal health outcomes. Collaboration fosters a sense of empowerment among patients, making them active participants in their care journey. This approach not only enhances patient's self-esteem but also encourages them to take ownership of their health, leading to improved compliance with treatment plans and overall wellness. Incorporating the theory of goal attainment into practice involves such a holistic approach to patient care.

Reflective Questions

1. Identify a problem you (or someone you know) may be experiencing/have a vested interest in resolving.
2. What is your anticipated approach to the problem?
3. What current information is needed, and where will you obtain this information?
4. What resources are needed (time, money, people)?
5. What specific strategies have been identified in devising a plan of action?
6. What outcomes (realistic, measurable, time sensitive) are anticipated?
7. How will you carry out and evaluate your plan?
8. What will you do with these findings?

Scenario

Integrating Theory and Evidence-Based Practice: The Nursing Process

John is a widowed, retired 68-year-old long-distance truck driver diagnosed with hypertension, obesity, chronic knee pain, and osteoarthritis of the left knee. Living alone on a farm 10 miles outside of the city, John has always been independent. He has no living relatives. The nearest neighbor lives 5 miles away.

Scheduled for knee replacement surgery, John has attended preoperative appointments and his preoperative laboratory tests are completed. After surgery, John will be transferred to the sub-acute unit of the hospital for rehabilitation. He has been told by his orthopedic surgeon that, depending on his recovery, he should expect to remain in the hospital for 3–7 days. John states that he "will be fine" and "doesn't need any help once home."

In developing a plan of care for this patient:

1. What do you recognize as priority problems/needs?
2. Identify three short-term goals
3. Identify three long-term goals

4. Which members of the health care team will be involved in the plan of care?
5. What significant information must be included in the discharge teaching plan?

Food for Thought

Theory to Practice: Resilience in Heartbreak

Heartbreak is inevitable. Yet there is truth in the statement that "what does not kill you makes you stronger." The pain of heartbreak, ultimately, inspires us. Unfortunately, when we are in the midst of despair, we are certain it's the end of the world. Time, self-care, and sharing the event (when you can bear to) on your own terms, and to a trusted individual, are keys to survival. Burying grief eventually comes back to haunt us in the form of unhealthy coping behaviors.

As a young nurse, I thought I was immune to such sorrow, believing that I had to be strong for my patients. Experiencing heartbreak through their eyes, I felt my job was to quickly "fix" any problem to cure anyone and everybody. I discovered that, while I was adept at giving advice, I was as fallible as my patients in accepting and acting on that information.

In my experience with heartbreak, the pain is visceral. Your heart pounds, you cannot breathe, and your chest is on fire. When those symptoms finally abate, the real work comes with confronting the all-consuming sadness that remains. My impatient character did not prepare me for this feeling. It paralyzed me, preventing me from completing the "activities of daily life." This familiar phrase was repeated over and over in nursing school as a red flag in the care of vulnerable patients. The inability to carry out even the simplest daily activities of life can signify physical or psychological trauma.

Sleeping helped. From working nights, I rationalized, I could fall asleep the minute my head hit the pillow, even if the world was coming down on my head. In my case, getting out of bed and putting two feet on the floor each morning was the challenge. As a wife, mother, and wage earner, I had no choice. People were dependent on me. Would they notice that I was barely able to function? Who could I trust to tell that I was hurting? Would I make a mistake at work?

I knew that suppressing my feelings by concentrating on my immediate responsibilities was a temporary fix, and it did work for a bit. But I also remembered from nursing school that unresolved issues return at some point in the form of somatic symptoms. I recall studying Freud's premise that we are all "simmering teakettles." If we avoid dealing with heartbreak at some point in our lives, we cannot begin to recover. We "boil over." Eventually the trauma of heartbreak will spiral and surface, usually triggered from some benign event, crippling us when we least expect it. It may appear as an anxiety attack while driving, attending a crowded venue, or watching a program on television.

As a childbirth instructor, I found that the labor relaxation and breathing exercises I taught expectant couples helped me when these feelings appeared out of nowhere. Also, I found myself remembering the five stages of grief by Elisabeth Kübler-Ross (denial, anger, bargaining, depression, acceptance) therapeutic. With the help of a counselor, I realized I had been moving in and out of these stages. I needed to reach acceptance. This is very much an individual experience with no concrete timetable, no statute of limitations. It can take years of hard work, patience, and hope to come to a resolution. But knowing there can be a resolution inspires us to move forward.

By far, the best advice I ever received when surviving a broken heart was from a true friend: "one year from now, no matter what the outcome, you will be in a better place." She didn't care to rehash the painful details of the heartbreak but instead was invested in healing her friend's pain and suffering. The heartbreak may still be there, but it remains as a memory, serving to empower us on many levels. At some point, we can revisit the experience, having learned from what it meant and maybe even coming to value the lessons it provided.

References

Baptiste, D. (2023). Integrating nursing theory into evidence-based practice: Bridging the gap between research and patient-centered care. *Research & Reviews: Journal of Nursing and Health Sciences, 9*(4), 1–2. https://doi.org/10.4172/JNHS.2023.9.4.92

Heron, R. (2023). Imogene King's theory of goal attainment: Empowering nurses to facilitate patient wellness. *Journal of Nursing Health Science, 9* (5), 1–2.

Kübler-Ross, E. (1969). *On death and dying: What the dying have to teach doctors, nurses, clergy, and their own families.* Scribner.

Kübler-Ross, E., & Kessler, D. (2005). *On grief and grieving: Finding the meaning of grief through the five stages of loss*. Simon and Schuster

Ominyi, J., & Alabi, A. (2025). Enhancing evidence-based practice implementation in acute care: A qualitative case study of nurses' roles, interprofessional collaboration, and professional development. *The Canadian Journal of Nursing Research*, 8445621251351056. https://doi.org/10.1177/08445621251351056

Figure Credit

Fig. 4.1: Jamie Murphy, "Nursing Theory," *Transitions to Professional Nursing Practice*, Lumen Learning. Copyright © 2022 by Jamie Murphy (CC BY 4.0) at https://courses.lumenlearning.com/suny-delhi-professionalnursing/chapter/nursing-theory/.

■ CHAPTER 5

Communication and Culture

Our ability to reach unity in diversity will be the beauty and the test of our civilization.

—Mahatma Gandhi

Introduction

This chapter presents two critical incidents involving communication, behaviors, and cultural sensitivity in nursing practice. Concepts and content are supported by this writer's cultural experiences in nursing practice. Through a global narrative of medical missions to South Africa and Haiti, a self-reflection exercise, and a scenario highlighting the challenges and communication barriers associated with ethical dilemmas surfacing from cultural assumptions, the goal is to inspire the readers' examination of their own cultural awareness.

Cultural Awareness

Cultural awareness involves recognizing and appreciating the diverse differences and similarities among those individuals sharing a common identity. Awareness requires an analysis of our own cultural values, beliefs, and biases, and an understanding of how these aspects affect our insights and communication with others. Cultural awareness extends far beyond "knowing" about a particular group's ethnicity or their practices.

Individuals have complex identities formed by race, ethnicity, religion, socioeconomic status, gender identity, and health status. As caregivers, recognizing these factors is essential in providing informed, current, individualized, and equitable care. Cultural awareness is essential in mental health and substance use contexts, as it guides providers to recognize how culture shapes individuals' experiences, addresses the impact of stigma, activates support systems and resources and promotes the development of effective, culturally sensitive, inclusive treatment.

The term cultural "competence" assumes that the more knowledge we have about another culture, the greater the competence we will exhibit in practice. Such a description places a heavy burden of responsibility on providers to" know it all" about each patient's culture. Moreover, this "categorical knowledge" about a particular population can lead to bias, stereotyping, and the impression that there is an end point to becoming fully culturally competent (Khan, 2021). Ultimately, preconceived notions about certain cultural groups can lead to treatment disparities.

The term "cultural humility" focuses on self-reflection in acknowledging one's own biases as a dynamic and ongoing process. Self-reflection involves understanding the complexity of identities: "even in sameness there is difference" (Khan, 2021). A clinician, therefore, can never be fully "competent" about the ever-changing nature of the patient experience.

In the critical incident "Close to Home," cultural stigma related to mental illness and substance use is a major obstacle to seeking help, leading to shame, isolation, and reluctance to seek treatment. As well, different cultures may hold distinct viewpoints when seeking help for loved ones with mental health conditions and substance use disorders. This influences how individuals recognize and interpret symptoms, whether they seek support, and how they cope. Effective mental health and substance use treatment requires culturally responsive care. This means understanding and integrating clients' cultural beliefs, values, and experiences into treatment plans. Cultivating cultural humility helps nurses and other health care providers approach each individual patient as the "expert" on their own cultural background and experiences.

Critical Incident One

Close to Home

Throughout my nursing career, a few incidents have provided insight, and teachable moments, and solidified my desire to continue in this field. One event in particular happened recently while working a shift at the detox facility where I am employed. A woman in her 40s was admitted to our unit, seeking care for decades of opiate use. I was orienting with the charge nurse, feeling nervous because I knew the responsibility that fell on the charge nurses, but excited because I love learning new skills and interacting with patients. We visited the patient in her room for an initial assessment; she was noticeably underweight, her hair and skin unkempt, and her clothes soiled in what appeared to be dirt/mud. She had visible track marks and scars bilaterally. She denied having any family to call and came here with only the clothes on her back. She explained that the last time she sought treatment for opiates was 20 years ago; she has been living on the streets ever since. It was apparent that her withdrawal symptoms were increasing quickly as the minutes passed. She was fidgety and restless, continuously getting up from the bed to pace the room or hallway. She complained of joint pain and was physically rubbing certain areas of her body. Her eyes were tearing up, and her nose was running. The vital signs showed she was hypertensive and tachycardic. She asked us for medications to get relief from how she was feeling.

The charge nurse and I explained the process and assured her that as soon as the doctor can put in a x1 STAT dose of methadone, we will have her visit the medication nurse. We offered comfort medications in the meantime consisting of Bentyl, Zofran, clonidine, and cyclobenzaprine. At the time, the line for the medication room was long, and she expressed the need to lie down for a while. For the next hour, the patient returned numerous times to the nurses' station, asking about the methadone and attempting to get to the medication window for the other medications offered, but the wait was still lengthy. She confided in me, stating, "If I don't get this methadone, I will have to leave (AMA) to go use. I don't want to use, but I have to because I can't continue to feel like this." At this point, she was presenting with a labile mood and frustration. The charge nurse received confirmation that the x1 STAT dose of methadone was ordered. We approached her in the common room to give the update and noticed she was crying and more restless than she had initially presented. We walked her to the medication nurse, who, unfortunately, told the patient she needed to wait her turn in line. The patient started yelling profanities and made her way back to her room. I quickly went down to de-escalate the situation and found out what had happened. She expressed feeling angry, unheard, unworthy, and physically sick. She stated she wanted to leave. I apologized for her having to wait so long and empathized with her feelings of frustration. I asked her if she could give me just five more minutes, and I would personally bring the medications down to administer to her. She was hesitant but agreed.

Within 3 minutes, I returned to her room with her methadone dose and comfort medications. Thirty minutes later, I visited again to reassess her; this time, her demeanor had changed. She was calm and relaxed, and said, "Thank you for being so nice to me, even when I was yelling and swearing, which I am sorry for. I just felt terrible and assumed nobody cared because, in the past, I had nurses tell me to leave if I wanted to leave AMA, but you stuck with it and did everything you could to get me to stay. I have never had that before. If I had left, I would have used, and I don't know how many more times I can get away with that before it's my last time; I don't want to do it anymore." I offered to get her some shower supplies and clothes from the donations to change into, which she accepted. After her shower, she returned to the nurses' station again to thank me for my kindness. She stayed the entire 7-day admission requirement and moved on to further treatment.

This situation affected me personally because I was overcome with joy knowing she stayed the entire length of time and did not leave AMA. What she does not know is that 6 years ago, my mother unfortunately passed away from an overdose. Professionally, it was a reminder of why this is my career. This specific patient population can be challenging at times, but I continue through those tough times with empathy and kindness because you may never know the kind of impact you have on a patient.

The writer above cited Dorothy Johnson's "behavioral systems model" theory as closely correlating to her field of work as an addictions nurse. Johnson's theory describes people as behavioral systems consisting of subsystems working to achieve homeostasis. These subsystems include biological, psychological, and sociological factors. She articulates that homeostasis happens with acclimation to internal and external adversities. In her work (Johnson, 1943), the author described a nursing student recognizing that the body might be ill only because of some mental strain; the mental condition might be due to some factor in the social or economic background of the patient (Johnson, 1943). Johnson reports that care today should be more than merely alleviating symptoms of physical distress. It must be concerned with the mental, emotional, and social well-being of the patient, as well as their physical comfort (Johnson, 1943).

According to the nurse who relates this poignant experience, Johnson's theory directly applies to her work in addictions nursing. People are made up of many different parts, which define their uniqueness. People who suffer from addictions are still people. They have lived experiences and social backgrounds that have brought them down the path they are traveling. Regardless of whether or not the addiction started as a choice or not, it has brought them to a state of hopelessness and despair. Many times, addiction continues because of a maladaptive way of coping with life. From a young age, these less-than-adequate coping skills were molded by taught behaviors, traumas, survival instincts, and belief systems. Treating a patient's physical condition is part of the nursing role. Providing safe and empathic patient-centered care is crucial to treating the social and emotional aspects of the patient, giving hope for the longevity of a patient's well-being.

Critical Incident Two

Culturally Congruent Nursing Care

My critical incident involves aspects of patient advocacy, cultural sensitivity, and equitable care related to a policy in a prenatal clinic in Africa. The policy identified that priority during clinic days would be given to women who attended the clinic with their partners or children's fathers. There were many women waiting to be served at the clinic. This policy would advantage only those who arrived with their partners. Women who were alone, their partners home caring for other children, as well as single mothers, had longer wait times, despite arriving early. The idea behind the policy was to get more men included in the pregnancy journey, foster support of their partners, and increase their involvement in the care of the newborn. However, this practice increased wait times for women who were alone. It was unfair and discriminatory. Most of the women had to sacrifice a whole day of work—and consequently wages—to be there. For those with partners, it was unfathomable that both sacrifice their day of work to attend clinics. Additionally, the clinic served women from different cultures; in some cultural groups, pregnancy is the concern of the woman and not the man. The policy favored women with partners who could afford to skip a day of work, such as those in formal employment, and it also favored women married to men who were allowed to actively attend prenatal clinics.

As nurses in the community, we challenged the policy and showed how it was unfair to those women. We collaborated to advocate for the single women who often had more burdens, such as having to find childcare for other children and living on one income. Moreover, we argued that for patients from certain cultures, the men would never come. Due to our patient advocacy, the clinic returned to a first-come, first-served basis, which allowed more women to plan their day. This experience had a profound personal and professional impact on me. Personally, I learned the importance of expressing oneself in building confidence. Professionally, it helped many disadvantaged people in the clinic. The policy was dangerous; it would seriously impact health-seeking behaviors for women from those cultural groups. From this experience, I make it a point in assessing patients to incorporate a person's culture and how this may impact their care.

This nurse in this scenario credits Leininger's culture care theory (Petiprin, 2019) in recognizing the importance of "culturally congruent care" for all patient populations. In her nursing career, Leininger identified a lack of knowledge in understanding the many variations required in patient care in order to support compliance, healing, and wellness. Leininger's theory attempts to provide culturally congruent nursing care through "cognitively based assistive, supportive, facilitative, or enabling acts or decisions that are mostly tailor-made to fit with individual, group's, or institution's cultural values, beliefs, and lifeways." The intent of the care is to fit with or have beneficial meaning and health outcomes for people of different or similar cultural backgrounds (Petiprin, 2019).

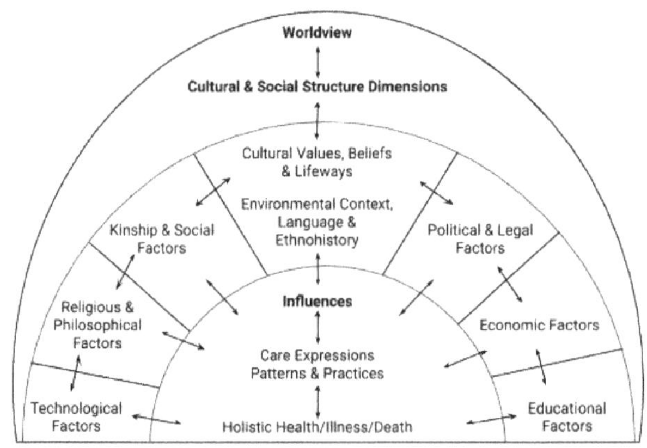

Figure 5.1 Leininger's Theory of Culture Care: Diversity and Universality
Created by Brian Duphily

Additionally, applicable to this case is nurse theorist Martha Elizabeth Rogers's "science of unitary human beings." Rogers asserts that nursing is both a science and an art; as such, nursing should provide care for the human being who is one with the environment. The science of nursing is the knowledge required by nurses to practice, while the art of nursing is the use of this knowledge to develop creative strategies to care for the patient (Razoni & Baker, 2023). The theory shows that a person cannot be separated from their environment. The nursing process based on the theory involves assessment, voluntary and mutual sharing, and evaluation. The assessment part would have helped prevent the described advocacy incident, as Rogers recommends a holistic assessment. This would include assessing the patient's employment status, income, marital, or partner status before developing such a policy. The nursing theory ensures that the nurse has complete information about a patient to allow for progression to the next step of the process, which involves sharing knowledge, provision of choices, and patient empowerment. For example, rather than implementing such a policy, patient education based on evidence and incorporating cultural needs should be done to encourage fathers to attend prenatal care (Walsh et al., 2021). The science of unitary human beings could help in such a situation in ensuring equitable care.

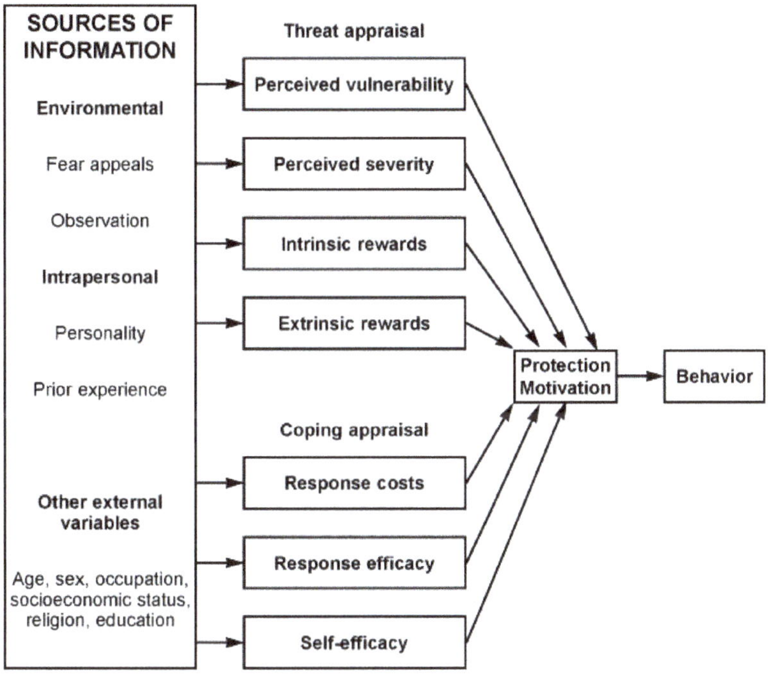

Figure 5.2 The Science of Unitary Human Beings Model

Food for Thought

Oh the Places You'll Go...as a Nurse

A Ripple in the Pond

Let us give publicity to HIV/AIDS and not hide it, because the only way to make it appear like a normal illness like TB, like cancer, is to come out and to say that somebody has died because of HIV.

—Nelson Mandela (2005)

In my career, I have had the good fortune to travel to different countries. In 2004, as a nurse, lactation consultant, and delegate of President Dwight Eisenhower's People-to-People Ambassador Program, I had the opportunity to visit South Africa with other program volunteers to work with mothers and babies diagnosed with/at risk for HIV.

Over the course of a few weeks in South Africa, I experienced first-hand the "ripple in the pond" effect. Working in the communities, baby sanctuaries, and hospitals, alongside the local, unsung heroes from Johannesburg and Cape Town facing the HIV/AIDS crisis was inspirational and humbling. The grass roots efforts of staff, family members, and volunteers made a difference every day.

Everyone we met invited us into their homes and their communities. They thanked us for coming "from so far away" and were grateful that we cared enough to help. It was usually the little things that counted. The children in particular were more impressed with the donations of soap, clothing, toothpaste, and towels, than in the baseball hats, stuffed animals, and toy trucks we brought to them in the Baby Sanctuary and orphanages.

We toured the prison at Robben Island, where Nelson Mandela spent 27 years for his political beliefs. Former political prisoners themselves, our tour guides showed us the limestone quarries where prisoners were given the arduous daily task of shoveling limestone from one corner of the quarry to the other, only to return it to its original site the following day. Mandela spent each day educating the other prisoners as they worked and invited the prison guards down from their posts to include them in the teaching sessions. This was the spirit of "reconciliation" that Mandela espoused.

Working in the clinic, we got to know the pregnant and post-partum mothers, who came daily to the center. While they waited for their appointment, they sang, made beautiful, beaded jewelry, and talked openly with us. Wearing "HIV positive" T-shirts, they were passionate and proud about their responsibility to educate others regarding the importance of early testing and care. The nurses shared the realities of working with little staff, of mothers who were formula feeding their babies with tainted water, and of children heading households. They rescued babies discarded in fields due to the stigma associated with the risk of HIV passed on to newborns, bringing them back from the edges of death. They spoke of the hope in the increasing availability of medicines for mothers and babies, of the pride they felt with the success of the Mothers Programmes, of Kangaroo Mother Care, and of the progress they began to see with more women seeking prenatal care and counseling.

From my trip to South Africa, I learned how the selfless activism of individuals not only raised awareness but effected positive behavior change in reducing HIV/AIDS transmission. I observed that no matter how desperate the situation, hope continues amid despair. These individuals speak of the future. I returned to the United States with the goal of spreading the word and found willing listeners. I was invited to speak (see the following speech) at churches, hospitals, schools, and local libraries. My audience members' overwhelming response was to support the Mothers Programmes with their donations. This innovative, grassroots program continues to thrive today (mothers2mothers, n.d.).

Speech and Newspaper Article

A Ripple in the Pond:

My Experience in South Africa

By Nancy Duphily

June 2005

Every 24 hours, it is estimated that over 2000 South Africans will be infected with the AIDS virus. Each year, one million babies are born in South Africa. Without treatment, over 25% of these mothers will transmit the virus to their babies, accounting for nearly 70,000 children born each year with the AIDS virus.

In just a decade, AIDS has progressed in South Africa from a tragic illness to an epidemic of historic proportions. Reading these statistics in a local newspaper about a country 16 hours by plane from Boston, one would think that South Africa is tragically doomed, that the figures are too high, and that there is little we can do, as individuals fighting our own personal daily battles.

Yet in my short journey to South Africa in November of 2004, I was constantly reminded of the "ripple in the pond effect." Seeing so many local unsung heroes in Johannesburg and Cape Town, educating, praying, nursing, and listening as they fight a daily battle to make a small dent in the HIV/AIDS crisis was an awe inspiring and humbling experience. They ARE making a difference, creating an impact. There is hope in the beautiful faces of the people who invited us into their homes and their communities. They thank us for coming and were genuinely impressed that we had come all the way from North America to see what we could do to help.

I remember feeling emotional and overwhelmed often here. It was usually the little things that would get to me. For example, the children at Cotlands Baby Sanctuary were more impressed with the gifts of soap, clothing, toothpaste, and towels, than in the baseball hats, stuffed animals, and toy trucks we brought to them in the orphanage. Another instance involved the perceptiveness of South Africans. Recognizing my Boston accent, Sowetans congratulated me on the Red Sox winning the World Series. I remember thinking, "Here we are, so many thousands of miles away, and few people own a television or radio, let alone electricity. This nation has survived years of violence and oppression. They are now facing 'the second apartheid' (as Bishop Desmond Tutu has dubbed the AIDS crisis). Life remains a daily struggle. Yet despite all of this, they took the time to recognize the success of the Boston Red Sox!"

The visit to Soweto's Hector Petersen Monument /Apartheid Museum was very powerful, with the recognition that in 1976, as we in the U.S. were celebrating 200 years of independence, children in South Africa were being killed for demanding freedom: the freedom of speech, the freedom to vote, and the freedom to be treated as an equal.

The visit to Robben Island, where Nelson Mandela was imprisoned for 27 years, was another moving experience. I wondered if I would sacrifice one quarter of my life for a belief I held so passionately. Tour guides, former political prisoners themselves, took us to the limestone quarries where prisoners were given the arduous daily task of shoveling limestone from one corner of the quarry to the other, only to return it to its original site the following day. Mandela spent each day educating the other prisoners as they worked, and soon invited the curious prison guards down from their posts to include them in the teaching sessions. Many were discharged from Robben Island with two advanced de3grees. This was the spirit of "reconciliation" that Mandela espoused. It is tragically ironic that Mandela recently lost his son, Makgatho, a 54-year-old lawyer, to AIDS.

The mothers of South Africa talked openly with us about their situations, let us take pictures freely, and never let their children out of their arms. There are no strollers, no playpens, and no car seats. Mothers keep their babies attached at all times. One mother said she never had a problem with infant diaper rash. She felt her little one squirming as she carried him on her back when he needed a diaper change. We admired the courage of the mothers, wearing "HIV positive" T-shirts, who are educating others regarding the importance of early testing and medical care.

The nurses escorted us to their hospitals and clinics, inside their neonatal intensive care units, their labor wards, and their baby sanctuaries. They were open and honest about the realities of working with no staff, of mothers formula-feeding their babies with tainted water, of children heading households, of rescuing discarded babies in a field to bring them back from the edges of death. They spoke of the hope in the increasing availability of medicines for mothers and babies, of the pride they felt with the success of the Mothers Programmes, of Kangaroo Mother Care, and of the progress they are seeing with more women seeking prenatal care and counseling.

My journey to South Africa has made me realize many things, one of which is that we are all in this together. As a global community, we share susceptibility. Yet we are not always in agreement. From working with people from Canada, Australia, South Africa, and other areas of the United States, I have learned to appreciate differences and the compromises we need to make if we are to create any impact on this pandemic.

Appreciating the differences of others is one thing. Education is another, but specific to this is in knowing your audience. Education happens everywhere. Our group saw this happening in the hospitals and clinics we visited through posters, songs, and peer support groups.

From my trip to South Africa, I have learned how the activism of individuals in helping to raise awareness, to change behavior and to create a positive response to the epidemic of HIV/AIDS in South Africa. I have observed in these people that no matter how desperate their situation, there is hope amidst the despair. They speak of the future.

*I feel my role is to become more educated, to care, and to continue the spirit of hope. This can be accomplished through communication. Spreading the word is vital with individuals, groups, and the communities here at home. We are not reminded daily of the pandemic "over there." We do not attend funerals daily for loved ones dying of HIV/AIDS. Spreading the word means assuring that people will not forget. One study estimated that 25 billion dollars a year could save 8 million lives annually. A small, charitable donation to Cotlands (*www.cotlands.org*) or to the Mothers Programmes (*www.mothersprogrammes.org*) are examples of honorable and civilized commitments to meet this challenge. We cannot let this epidemic win. In the words of Nelson Mandela, "Let us give publicity to HIV/AIDS and not hide it, because the only way to make it appear like a normal illness like TB, like cancer, is to come out and to say that somebody has died because of HIV."*

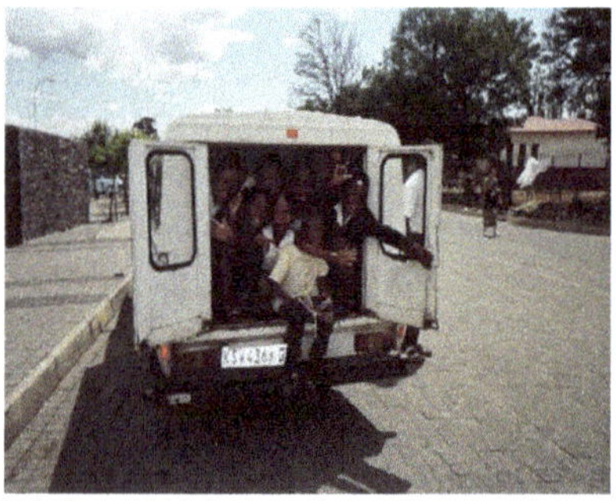

Image 5.1

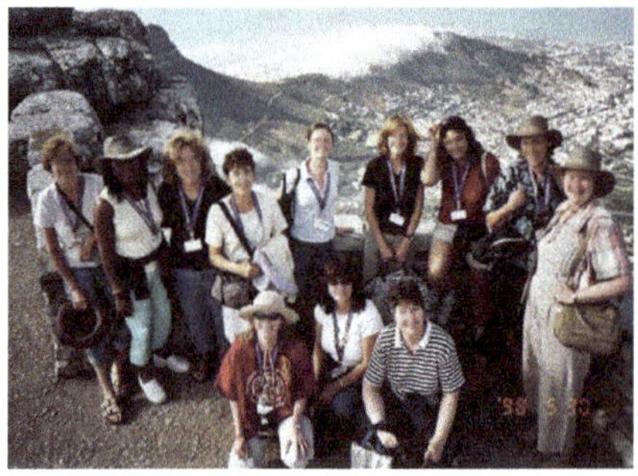

Image 5.2

Forward in Health Medical Mission Trip

Les Cayes, Haiti

We hear and read about poverty.

Until you are there and see it and breathe it and feel it and smell it, you really don't understand it.

—Dr. John Mulqueen

July 2007 presented the opportunity of a lifetime for 12 high school and college students, along with six medical professionals, who volunteered for a medical mission in Les Cayes, Haiti. Working in clinics, nursing homes, and orphanages in the community, my 16-year-old son Brian and I were part of this group. We spent 2 weeks there to help conduct a series of pediatric clinics providing free medical treatment to 277 children. The trip was organized by Forward in Health (FIH), a local nonprofit organization from Gardner, Massachusetts.

Under the direction of Dr. John Mulqueen and Paula Mulqueen, RN, FIH began organizing medical mission trips to Les Cayes, Haiti, following their attendance at a presentation by the Diocese of Worcester's Haitian Apostolate. Initial visits to bring much-needed medical care to Haiti gained so much community support that the Mulqueens were able to formally establish FIH as a nonprofit organization. During our trip to Les Cayes, FIH was preparing to build a permanent medical clinic on three acres of land, acquired with donations provided by an anonymous benefactor. Joining the Mulqueens and volunteers was "Roudy," FIH's on-site director in Haiti. His insights into citizens' needs, weather conditions, political unrest, and other critical factors were crucial in advising FIH on everything from urgent medical conditions to travel safety.

Our time with FIH involved working in pediatric clinics in three different locations within the southern region of Les Cayes. Dedicated to providing healthcare to Haiti's most needy citizens in this rural area, individuals worked 3 days at the clinics, visited the orphanage, held many babies, participated in a dance recital with local teens, and completed repair projects at a local nursing home. We were all were struck by the friendliness, pride, and resiliency of the Haitian people, despite overwhelming poverty and challenging living conditions. A typical family home is about the size of a one-car American garage, constructed of wood planks and a tin roof. Some homes lack electricity and plumbing; homeowners use wood or coal as a main source of fuel. Volunteers stayed at a comfortable "mission house," considered "palatial" by Haitian standards.

During our time in Les Cayes, it was noted that about half of the 277 children seen in the clinics were treated for intestinal parasites, upper respiratory infections, rashes, and ear infections. More serious conditions included heart problems and tuberculosis. In addition to the time spent administering direct care to patients, volunteers visited, played with, and helped care for children in the Haitian orphanage run by the Sisters of Charity, the order founded by Mother Teresa. All of the medications and supplies used in the clinics were either donated directly or paid for through charitable contributions to FIH. This organization worked diligently to raise the funds and resources needed to construct, furnish, and operate a permanent medical clinic, staffed by Haitian clinicians and community workers, on the plot of land recently purchased by the organization.

Somewhere in all of us, we seek help beyond our comfort zone. The most important thing you need with community service is passion. You need passion and you need compassion. We are not going to be able to save the world or save Haiti. We give the best possible care that we can give while we're there, whether it's 8 days or 2 weeks.

—Dr. John Mulqueen

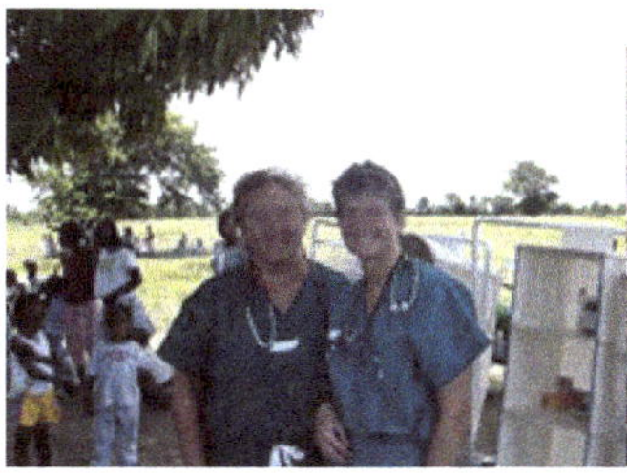
Image 5.3

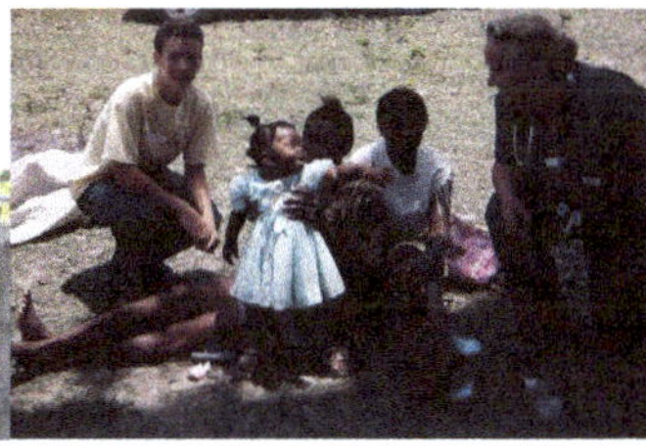
Image 5.4

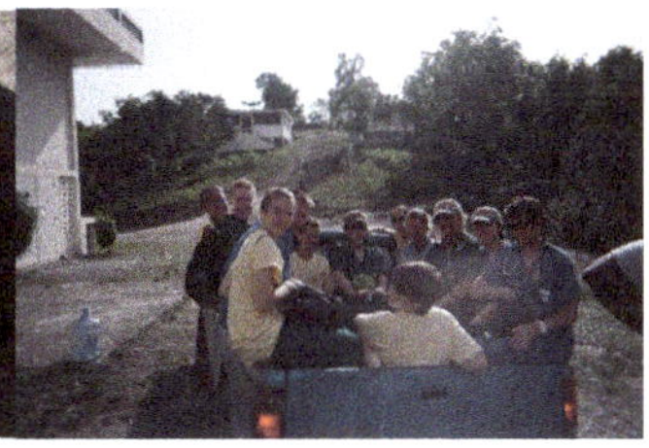
Image 5.5

Scenario

Communication, Culture, and Ethics

A non-English speaking female patient arrives alone in the emergency department. Through interpreter services, the triage nurse learns that the patient, a 34-year-old Haitian mother of three (ages 9, 5, and 2 years of age) has experienced epigastric pain, nausea, and vomiting for 36 hours. Diagnostic tests reveal findings of acute cholecystitis. The patient is scheduled for laparoscopic cholecystectomy. During the admission assessment the patient states that her family recently moved away from relatives and friends for her husband's new job opportunity here. She expresses concern about her partner's ability to care for her children and worries about how she will manage at home after discharge. The nurse offers to contact the patient's husband. Additionally, she places a request for a social service consult, suggesting a family meeting and visiting nursing services be arranged.

Reflective Questions

1. What assumptions are being made here?
2. What additional information is needed?
3. How might the ethical principles below assist the nurse to better assess and intervene in this situation?

    a. Autonomy
    b. Beneficence
    c. Fidelity
    d. Justice

References

Johnson, D. (1943). Learning to know people. *American Journal of Nursing, 43*(3), 248–252.

Khan, S. (2021, January 13).*Cultural humility vs. cultural competence—and why providers need both*. Boston Medical Center. https://healthcity.bmc.org/category/mental-health-and-addiction/

Mandela's eldest son dies of Aids. (2005, January 6). *The Guardian*. https://www.theguardian.com/world/2005/jan/06/southafrica.aids

mothers2mothers. (n.d.). *South Africa*. Retrieved January 11, 2006, from https://m2m.org/what-we-do/where-we-work/south-africa-2

Petiprin, A. (2019). *Leininger's culture care theory*. Nursing Theory. https://nursing-theory.org/theories-and-models/leininger-culture-care-theory.php

Razoni, S. A., & Baker, K. (2023). *Martha Rogers: Science of unitary human beings*. Nurseslabs. https://nurseslabs.com/martha-e-rogers-theory-unitary-human-beings/

Walsh, T. B., Carpenter, E., Costanzo, M. A., Howard, L., & Reynders, R. (2021). Present as a partner and a parent: Mothers' and fathers' perspectives on father participation in prenatal care. *Infant Mental Health Journal*, *42*(3), 386–399.

Figure Credits

Fig. 5.1: Generated using Google Gemini.

Fig. 5.2: S. Sutton, "Health Behavior: Psychosocial Theories," *International Encyclopedia of the Social & Behavioral Sciences*, https://www.sciencedirect.com/science/chapter/referencework/abs/pii/B0080430767038729. Copyright © 2001 by Elsevier B.V.

■ CHAPTER 6

Civility

Be civil to all, sociable to many, familiar with few, friend to one, enemy to none.

—Benjamin Franklin

Introduction

Civility is defined as respectful engagement when differing opinions or opposing views are expressed in order to promote community, the common good, and meaningful connections. This definition implies proactive behaviors displayed during difficult events, voicing one's opinion while supporting others. It is the sum of compromises individuals make to live harmoniously in society. Differences are resolved in a respectful ways (Clark, 2022).

Incivility in the profession is demonstrated in this first critical incident with the author's depiction of workplace violence concerns. Complex and multifaceted, these situations can exceed the limits of a nurses' duty to provide care. In the "strengths-based nursing" account, the author "shifts" her thinking to strategize interventions to meeting the patient's ongoing needs, while maintaining her safety.

Vulnerability is a crucial element in determining the safety risks a nurse faces at the hands of a potentially violent patient. Also, the vulnerabilities of the patient as the recipient of care are determined based on their dependency on this care, and their capacity to appreciate the impacts of their actions. These vulnerabilities impact the strength of the provider's "duty to provide care" (Dunsford, 2022) in the face of personal risk.

The nurse in Critical Incident Two exemplifies the definition of civility: "proactive behaviors displayed during difficult events" (Clark et al., 2021). This is evidenced through a surgical nurse orientee's eyes as two trauma cases appear simultaneously in the operating room. In this event, the writer observes clear role expectations and collaboration, as well as the surgical team's mutual respect for one another. Controlled chaos was maintained in an atmosphere of civility and professionalism, created and role modeled among members of the health care team.

Critical Incident One

Civility Through the Lens of "Strengths-Based" Nursing

Workplace violence comprises part of my role as a home care nurse. Staying safe in a family's home can be especially tricky and involves an extreme amount of finesse. I can deliver the best textbook clinical care, according to the designated plan, to a patient. The family, who typically observes me on their loved one's care, may find some minutia of fault. While I understand the stress that families undergo in the daily complex care of a family member, I feel the reality of nurses as lightning rods for their ire. I have learned to always have my keys and phone on me after being cornered in a room on an overnight shift for giving a father's son oxygen when the boy's oxygen saturation level was 88%. As a homecare nurse, I am often judged by people who are not nurses and have no idea just how hard we work to become one. I recognize that hospitals are stretched thin, along with the reality that families may not have experienced comprehensive discharge education for their loved one. Agencies stressing "better customer service skills" downplay these safety issues, which present barriers in building an alliance with the family. How can I teach evidenced-based practice (EBP) care when "the hospital didn't do it like that"?

This nurse found answers in the book *Strengths-Based Nursing Care: Health and Healing for Person and Family* (Gottlieb, 2012).

After a particularly bad day at work, I "recalibrate" by reviewing a particular section of Gottlieb's book relevant to my experience. This author helped me look at the family as a component of what is going right and become more effective as a team member. Using the "strengths-based nursing care goggles" teaches me that, while I may give great care to a patient, the family is the gatekeeper allowing me in the home. While I still have my "WWFD?" (What would Flo do?) Florence Nightingale moments, Gottlieb delivers the words to guide me in my current daily practice. I have learned that homecare is never about just one patient. I now recognize the value of including the support of family in the journey of caring for a medically fragile patient in their home.

Building on Nightingale's theory, author Laurie Gottlieb's philosophy emphasizes "Good News"—that is, what is "going right" and starting from there to implement positive changes at the appropriate time. Florence Nightingale believed that nurses could encourage or discourage the healing process based on their interactions with a patient. Nurses who attempted to falsely cheer up a patient were not creating an environment conducive to healing. Good news, she proposed, could assist a patient in becoming healthier.

Nightingale also encouraged nurses to examine their patient's social networks (Riegel et al., 2021). Having close family or friends near to the patient, although sometimes a challenge, would improve the environment for the patient. With the goal of nursing to eradicate an illness, Nightingale believed that nurses should heed what was being said by visitors and encourage positive interactions. Her environmental theory of nursing focuses on patient care. By individualizing each patient's environment, healing could be created and deeper relationships between the patient and nurse (and family) could form. In this way, the best care possible could be provided.

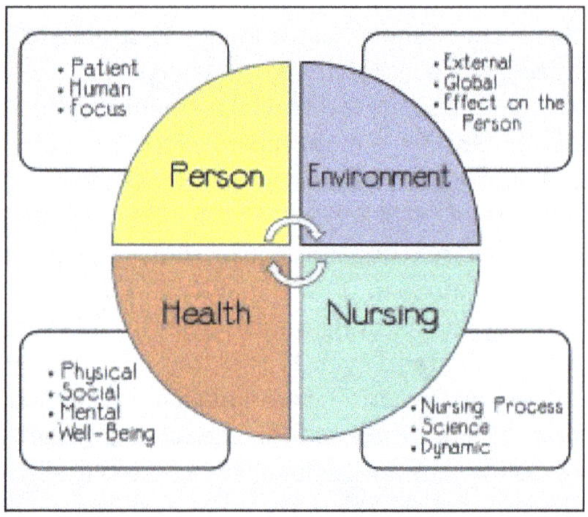

Figure 6.1 Person, Environment, Nursing, and Health

Critical Incident Two

Civility in Controlled Chaos

I was at the beginning of my nursing orientation in the operating room and two traumas appeared at the exact same time. Both traumas were unrelated stabbings coming into the operating simultaneously for exploratory laparotomies. I assisted with one of the traumas. Adrenaline was flowing through all members of the care team as we set up the room with instruments, pulled medications, set up a cell saver to filter and reuse blood, and gathered additional blood from the blood bank to transfuse during surgery. I felt a profound sense of pride and accomplish-

ment. I saw the whole surgical team work together to prepare for these patients and maintain their stability. I felt like I was effective with my preparation and assistance to others through the situation. Anyone receiving help that afternoon was grateful, whether it meant running for supplies, inserting a Foley, to transfusing blood. The aftermath of working thorough the stress of a traumatic situation can be just as rewarding when the outcome is positive. This critical incident reinforced why I chose nursing in the first place. This was a day I will truly never forget.

A nursing theory that parallels the care and interventions caried out in this critical incident can be seen in Faye Abdellah's "Twenty-One Nursing Problems," which focuses on meeting the physical, social, and emotional needs of the individual patient in assessment, nursing diagnosis, and planning interventions. The ultimate goal in applying this theory is achievement of optimum health by using a patient-centered approach. All aspects of the patient's well-being should be considered when assessing and making a nursing diagnosis. Abdellah's theory consists of 10 steps to identify the patient's issues, and eleven skills used to create a nursing plan from data obtained (Mudd et al., 2020). Abdellah believed that nurses should help meet the patient's needs from a basic to a more complex level approach (Mehraeen et al., 2020).

Table 6.1 Ten Steps to Identify the Patient's Problem

1. Learn to know the patient.
2. Sort out relevant and significant data.
3. Make generalizations about available data in relation to similar nursing problems present by other patients.
4. Identify the therapeutic plan.
5. Test generalizations with the patient.
6. Validate the patient's conclusions.
7. Continue to observe and evaluate the patient over a period of time to identify any attitudes and clues affecting his or her behavior.
8. Explore the patient and his or her family's reactions to the therapeutic plan and involve them in the plan.
9. Identify how the nurses feel about the patient's nursing problems.
10. Discuss and develop a comprehensive nursing plan.
Source: Adapted from Faye Abdellah, "10 Steps to Identify the Patient's Problem," Patient-Centered Approaches to Nursing, https://nurseslabs.com/wp-content/uploads/2014/08/Faye-Abdellah-10-Steps.png. Copyright © 1960 by Macmillan.

Reflective Questions

1. Have you experienced incivility, bullying, or workplace violence?
2. What was your response?
3. What policies or resources exist in your workplace that foster civility?

4. How can you contribute to help build and maintain positive a civil work environment?
5. How can you improve your communication and conflict-negotiation skills to address incivility?

Scenario

Incivility and Workplace Violence

As an associate's degree in nursing (ADN) graduate with 5 years' experience, Jillian spent most of her previous career working on a subacute unit of a 200-bed hospital in her city. Three years ago, Jillian enrolled part time in an RN to BSN program at a local university, graduating with honors. Now employed as a staff RN on a medical surgical unit, she began completing a 6-week orientation.

Jillian maintained a positive working relationship with her preceptor, who was assigned consistently to Jillian for 1 month. Because of a medical emergency, her preceptor was now unavailable. During the last 2 weeks of her orientation, the hospital's director of nursing education found a replacement in Ivy, an RN on the same unit for over 10 years, who precepted a new graduate once before, a year ago.

Ivy told Jillian that she was "assigned" to the preceptor role and voiced her concerns about the "extra work" involved. Her statements, "There is no way you can get a BSN in that short amount of time," and "What kind of a program are they running over there at the university?," worried Jillian. Although still on orientation, Jillian was left alone to make her own decisions. A conflict occurred when Jillian overlooked a client's confusion and fall, attributed to a newly prescribed medication. Ivy angrily reprimanded Jillian at the nurses' station. Jillian felt overwhelmed and defeated and considered resigning from the position: "Maybe my nursing program did not prepare me...maybe my original preceptor was too easy on me."

You are the nurse manager of the unit charged with resolving this situation.

- How do the factors cited in the title of this scenario contribute to this scenario?
- Are there additional factors that come into play?
- How might this situation have been avoided?
- What strategies and resources should be in place at this time?

Food for Thought

An Early Lesson in Civility

This story takes place in the 1960's, during a family summer trip from Rhode Island to Niagara Falls. My father had a new 1959 Chevy Impala, and he wanted to test it out. Per the usual seating arrangements, my parents and oldest sister were riding in front. The "next" eldest were the "twins" (as they would be called all of their lives), who were in the back, each scoring a window seat. As the youngest child in 1960, I was relegated to the middle of the back seat, wedged in between my sisters' sharp elbows jabbing me in the ribs. There was no hope of any "window time." I sought my revenge by continuously bugging them, whining quietly in their ears so my father would not hear. This always got them going. We silently fought the whole way.

At one point, one of the twins hung her doll clothes on the hook over her window. With no air conditioning in the car, the windows were fully down, and my father was flying along the highway. Minutes later, the doll's ensemble flew out and disappeared somewhere along the Mohawk Trail. My sister let out a howl to stop, but my dad, not happy at even a suggestion that we might sabotage his travel time, continued on, yelling, "Too bad … you won't do that again!" We had miles to go and, at this point, were just entering the "Hairpin Turn." The doll clothes were seen drifting to the bottom of the Mohawk Valley below us.

There were few four-lane highways back in the 1960's, so automobile trips took a bit longer. My mother told us we would break up the ride by "staying in a hotel." I heard my parents saying it would cost us $9.00 a night (for the six of us). The "hotel" turned out to be two rustic cabins from something out of Grimm's Fairy Tales, complete with spiders and weird smells.

My parents took us out to a restaurant that night. My Dad told us we could have anything we wanted on the menu. All of us ordered steak and a Shirley Temple (ginger ale and grenadine, topped off with a maraschino cherry). Fancy! We thought this was the greatest adventure ever, and we hadn't even arrived at Niagara Falls yet.

Because the trip was long, my mother packed a huge cardboard box of crayons and enough paper to last the 500-mile trip. When we arrived, we were done with coloring. We bounded out of the car to see what Niagara Falls, and its sights, had to offer. We stored the huge crayon box in the back seat window (of our brand-new 1959 Chevy Impala).

Hours later, we returned to the car to find a kaleidoscope of color in the back seat. In the hot August sun, the crayons had all melted together into a congealed rainbow of colored wax, cascading down the back seat of my father's new ride. Scrub as we might, we never really got rid of that crayon residue. We ended up putting a blanket over the mess. I think I have blotted out from my memory my father's reaction, but I am pretty sure it was also colorful. I also do not remember how long we kept that car, but what I do recall was a very quiet trip home.

References

Clark, C. M., Gorton, K. L., & Bentley, A. L. (2022). Civility: A concept analysis revisited. *Nursing Outlook, 70*(2), 259–270. https://doi.org/10.1016/j.outlook.2021.11.001

Dunsford, J. (2022). Nursing violent patients: Vulnerability and the limits of the duty to provide care. *Nursing Inquiry, 29*(2), e12453. https://doi.org/10.1111/nin.12453

Gottlieb, L. (2012). *Strengths-based nursing care: Health and healing for person and family.* Springer Publishing Company.

Gottlieb, L. (2014). Strengths-based nursing, a holistic approach to care, grounded in eight core values. *American Journal of Nursing, 114*(8) 24–32.

Mehraeen, P., Nazarpour, P., & Ghanbari, A. (2020). Designing a nursing care plan based on Faye Glenn Abdellah model in patients with diabetes type 2: A case study. *International Journal of Caring Sciences, 13*(3), 2250–2260.

Mudd, A., Feo, R., Conroy, T., & Kitson, A. (2020). Where and how does fundamental care fit within seminal nursing theories: A narrative review and synthesis of key nursing concepts. *Journal of Clinical Nursing, 29*(19–20), 3652 3666. https://doi.org/10.1111/jocn.15420

Riegel, F., Crossetti, M.D.G.O., Martini, J. G., & Nes, A.A.G. (2021). Florence Nightingale's theory and her contributions to holistic critical thinking in nursing. *Revista brasileira de enfermagem, 74*(2), e20200139. https://doi.org/10.1590/0034-7167-2020-0139

Figure Credit

Fig. 6.1: Jamie Murphy, "Nursing Theory," *Transitions to Professional Nursing Practice*, Lumen Learning. Copyright © 2022 by Jamie Murphy (CC BY 4.0) at https://courses.lumenlearning.com/suny-delhi-professionalnursing/chapter/nursing-theory/.

■ CHAPTER 7

Lifelong Learning

Wisdom is not a product of schooling but of the lifelong attempt to acquire it.

—Albert Einstein

Introduction

Lifelong learning, also known as continuing professional development (CPD), informs nurses' knowledge and skills. When maintained alongside a supportive working environment, CPD ultimately leads to improved patient care standards, attitudes, and motivation. A lifelong learning approach signifies the value that providers place in upholding high standards of care through competent practice (Mlambo et al., 2021).

The critical incidents included in Chapter 7 demonstrate that lifelong learning, coupled with the clinical experience and intuition it imparts, supports, and guides significant changes and approaches to the care nurses provide. More a "gut feeling," intuition is a process based on the knowledge and care experience that has a place beside research-based evidence. Nurses integrate both analysis and synthesis of intuition alongside objective data when making decisions. Integrating intuition into clinical practice supports decision-making, which increases the quality and safety of patient care (Melin-Johansson et al., 2017).

Critical Incident One

"Still Learning": Intuition in the Resource Nurse Role

Nursing encompasses an art, a humanistic orientation, a feeling for the value of the individual, and an intuitive sense of ethics, and of the appropriateness of action taken.

—Myrtle Aydelotte, PhD, RN, FAAN

I work with pediatric families who deal with the most unimaginable: their child is diagnosed with cancer. Some families cope well in these unfair circumstances, but other families struggle considerably. They can be unable to cope emotionally, financially, and sometimes intellectually. A pediatric cancer diagnosis is not only a diagnosis for the child (patient) but encompasses and affects the entire family. My job is to meet the patients and families where they are (emotionally, intellectually) while providing the best care. For each patient, I also have moms, dads, brothers, and sisters to consider in this primary care practice. Even after 20 years in nursing, I am nervous when covering for another nurse in caring for one of their patients. Our clinic is small enough that we are all versed in every patient's diagnosis and treatment. This past week, we had a particularly busy day in the clinic, and I was the "resource nurse." Every nurse had a busy assignment, and two challenging patients (primary patients of my coworker on maternity leave) were scheduled. I made the assignment in the morning, leaving these two patients unassigned.

As the day progressed I quietly decided as a resource nurse to just step up and take the patients as they arrived. One was an 8-year-old just off treatment for acute myelogenous leukemia (AML), who was extremely emotional and unable to cope during her treatment. Her clinic visits historically were long and draining. Needless to say, I was intimidated caring for her. I approached her with a positive and can-do attitude. Her IV access and therapeutic phlebotomy went as smoothly as possible. She left feeling proud of herself for coping well.

I was relieved, just in time for the second patient, diagnosed with rhabdomyosarcoma. He was in the clinic for a disconnect from hydration, de-access of a port-a-cath, Neulasta® injection, and the cherry on top—a rabies injection (he had been exposed to a bat). He is unable to cope with most interventions, so knowing I had four to accomplish was daunting. I approached with the same cheerful outlook, and all tasks were completed in a caring manner. He too left the clinic smiling, and again, I was relieved

All of these years later, I am still learning, particularly knowing when as a leader to delegate, when to step up, and when to bear the burden. I could see that we were drowning in patient care. Every nurse was challenged with the care they were providing. I took the two unassigned patients and completed the work.

Even after 20 years in the profession, I am learning to lean into my experience. I am finding there is a time to rely on experience gained and a time to learn. Neither of these patients had complex care. They were simple tasks in theory but still felt overwhelming because of how the patient might react to my actions. I trusted myself and chose not to let the challenge daunt me. My colleagues were grateful, not even realizing that the patients had been cared for while ifosfimide, etoposide, rituximab, bleomycin, vinblastine (to name a few) were infusing with other patients. It may seem like a small issue (in its nature and outcome), but it was meaningful to me.

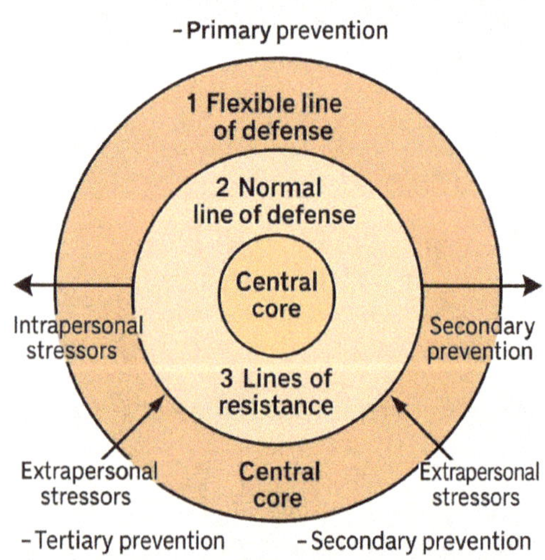

Figure 7.1 Betty Neuman's Systems Model

In this critical incident, Betty Neuman's "systems model" is applied to with respect to the stressors posed and the response displayed. The incident exemplifies the need for a holistic approach to nursing situations and flexibility within care. The nurse in this scenario takes a step back from the situation itself. Based on her education, experience, and expertise, she reassesses her approach and develops an individualized plan for the patient and family in a way that meets their particular needs.

The Neuman systems model is based on the person's relationship to stress, response, and reconstituting factors that are progressive in nature. As a holistic system-based method in nursing that maintains flexibility, it focuses on patient's responses to environmental stressors while utilizing primary, secondary, and tertiary prevention methods to reduce stressors (Montano, 2021). Neuman believed there was a constant exchange of energy in patient environments, and this exchange was made up of many interrelated parts.

Nurses promote patients' defenses through role modeling, education, emotional support, and resources related to their specific needs. By capitalizing on these strengths, we help patients build stress resilience, which is key for overall health. Additionally, this nurse recognizes her own stress triggers. As seen in the previous story, taking the time to pause and regain balance fosters one's own need to be emotionally stable in order to effectively support others.

Intuition

Another important skill that plays a key role in this critical incident concerns the "skill" of intuition. Intuition is the ability that nurses employ, but seldom outwardly consider, in clinical practice. Understanding intuition and its application in healthcare ensures high-quality, safe patient care. Most nurses will label intuition as a "gut feeling" (Hassani et al., 2016) used to supplement the decision-making process.

Intuition does not operate in a vacuum. It is incorporated into a nurse's assessment skills, combined with years of experience, expertise, and a fundamental foundation from entry level nursing education. Intuition helps the nurse to recognize patterns in their practice and those similarities that occur among workplace experiences. Changes in patient behaviors and the feeling that "something is not right" often prompt further investigation and intervention (Benner & Tanner, 1987).

Intuition allows nurses to process, order, and prioritize relevant information among the host of additional factors that nurses recognize in their assessment and plan in patient care. Benner and Tanner (1987) report that intuition helps nurses to engage with a of unstructured situations, where the existing "cookbook" of tools or guidelines may be less than useful. During this time, however, the nurse may be applying intuition without explicitly articulating what they are doing. This may explain why nurses with more years of clinical experience are more likely to report that they rely on a sense of intuition when making decisions in practice than in other forms of knowledge (i.e., seeking out evidence via research articles, collaboration with other providers).

Authors Anton et al. (2021) agree that the nurse's prior experience in handling previous situations influences their intuition. Nurses use this wealth of knowledge in conjunction with clinical skills to assess and plan decisions in patient care. This experience may help nurses to subconsciously identify patterns that have surfaced in previous patient events to inform their decisions and subsequently initiate timely intervention.

Turan et al. (2019) identified that a nurse's level of emotional intelligence of recognition and management of emotions surrounding them can contribute to the use of intuition in clinical decision-making. Emotional intelligence has been associated with increased levels of self-awareness, perception, and effective communication skills, valuable tools in recognizing and diagnosing patients' needs.

Ensuring that nurses are empowered to build on their intuitive abilities is a significant element of health care practice to be considered. Measuring these proficiencies can be daunting given the complex array of factors involved, which may hinder identification of strategies for nurses in developing their intuitive strengths. Further research into the role of intuition is essential in order to strategize methods to improve patient care.

Critical Incident Two

Role Modeling: "It Was the Nurses"

When I was pregnant with my twins, I was on bedrest for 55 days due to premature rupture of membranes (PROM). Those days were mostly uneventful, but one night around 11:30 pm I started having cramps that were a worse than usual, but I thought they were nothing. I told the nurse and she was so calm and thorough while she cared for me and notified the doctor, and she really got the ball rolling when the doctor did an exam and said, "We gotta go now." I don't remember everything about that night because I ended up being a code white emergency C-section due to placental abruption, and the last thing I remember was a team rushing me to the OR and there were so many people there and I can best describe it as organized chaos. There was yelling and there was rushing, but it was orchestrated perfectly. My nurse's calmness and professionalism were top notch, and she did everything she could to make sure I was comfortable and called my husband and kept him informed of everything until he could get to the hospital. I remember waking up around 3 in the morning while the nurses were wheeling myself in my bed into the NICU and moving things around so I could see my babies, and at that point the doctor told me one of my twins was not going to make it. I had told the nurse beforehand whatever happens and whatever my babies looked like, I wanted to see them no matter what. The nurses were so kind and compassionate and did everything they could to get me to the NICU quickly. The outcome of this event was the best case scenario, against all odds my daughter pulled through and is now 7 and thriving. This event affected me personally, and when working with parents, I have so much compassion for families and do everything I can to put their preferences first and ensure that families have information and are involved and patients are empowered to be in charge of their own care.

The nursing theorist I feel most strongly relates to my experience is Watson's caring theory; the nurse had established a caring relationship, but she also fostered team relationships, coordinated care, and was "authentically present." You could tell this nurse really cared and wasn't just there for the money or the prestige. Watson's theory focuses on patient-centered care and a method of caring for patients that works with them while they attain or maintain health. The caring theory includes coordinating care, communicating the plan of care, utilizing the nursing process, encouraging patient and team relationships, promoting professional excellence, and communicating the plan of care, among outside tenets such as involving community resources and incorporating evidence-based practice

The nurse on shift that night utilized the nursing process and was methodical in her exam of me, thorough of her prepping me for surgery, and watching the fetal monitor while also being caring and compassionate knowing that she was dealing with a life-or-death situation.

This nurse identifies Jean Watson as the nurse theorist who sums up what she is feeling about her experience and how it changed her. Watson defines nursing as an independent role with unique disciplines and values that impact patients (Ghanbari-Afra, et al., 2022). Watson explains that her caring theory is based on the fact that humans should be treated as themselves, others, and nature, not as objects. While in the NICU, this future nurse was treated as an integral part of the team. She played a part in her son's care while the nurses cared for them both.

The work of Kristen Swanson (1991) applies in this setting, as well. Dr. Swanson's caring model emphasizes the importance of building therapeutic relationships in patient care. Her theory emphasizes the importance of universal, person-centered care that considers the physical, emotional, and spiritual needs of individuals. In her work, Swanson focuses on a range of ideas in the caring process: maintaining belief, knowing, being with, doing for, and enabling, all of which guide nurses in forming meaningful connections with patients, and lead to providing holistic, individualized, effective nursing care (Alligood, 2022).

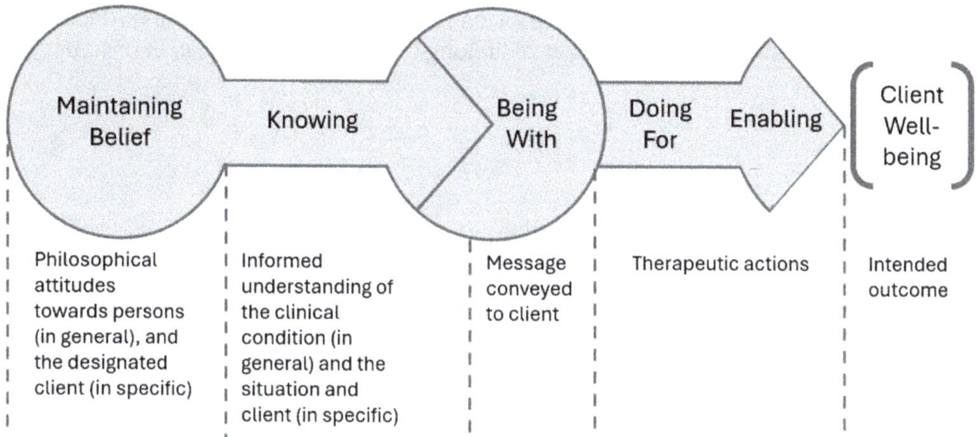

Figure 7.2 The Structure of Caring

Reflective Questions

1. How would you define "lifelong learning"?
2. Would you describe yourself as a lifelong learner? Why?
3. What are some of the advantages of lifelong learning?
4. What roles do factors such as self-motivation, reading, curiosity, and career planning play in one's pursuit of lifelong learning?
5. How might an individual develop a lifelong learning "mindset"?

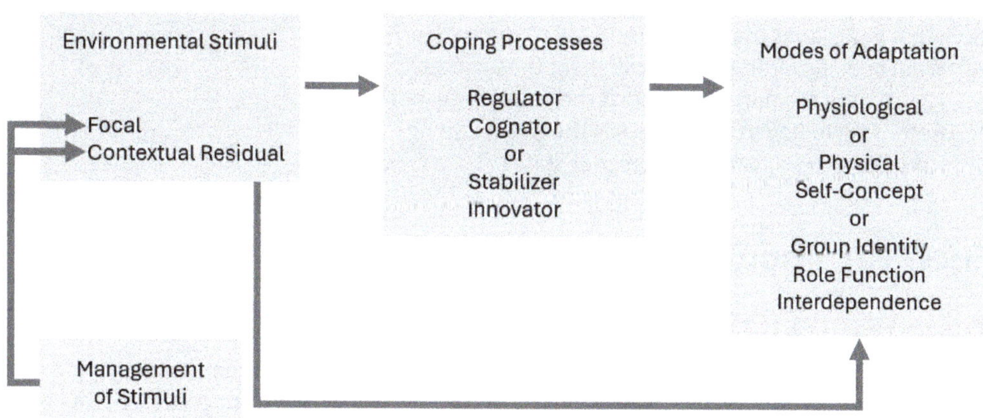

Figure 7.3 The Roy Adaption Model
Created by Brian Duphily

Introduction to the Scenario

Sister Callista Roy's adaptation model addresses human beings as holistic adaptive systems that constantly change and interact with their environment (Roy, 2009). Health is the process of being and becoming integrated and reflects both environment and person. Roy's adaptation model focuses on four life "processes": physiologic, self-concept, role function, and interdependence modes. In this scenario, the focus is on role function, coping, and interdependence as nurses embrace the important concept of lifelong learning in adapting to informatics technology.

Scenario

Nurses use the "FLOW" electronic health record (EHR) system at Fremont General. The assessment portion evaluates each client using a systems approach similar to nursing theorist Callista Roy's adaptation model, and the first level of assessment: physiologic-physical mode, where nurses assess and note items such as oxygenation, safety, and level of neurological functioning. Care plans are updated each shift and include areas such as the client's disposition, safety, and nutritional needs. A "free text" section allows for documentation of individual client-specific issues. The method of approach to this section utilizes Roy's model, where nursing diagnoses (problems), patient-specific interventions and goals, and means of evaluation are listed.

A recently widowed 70-year-old patient arrives at the ED with shortness of breath (SOB) related to a medical diagnosis of congestive heart failure (CHF). He has stopped taking his prescribed Lasix medication, stating it makes him urinate frequently. He reports that since his wife has died, he takes most of his meals at local fast-food restaurants.

Reflection

1. In completing the patient assessment/EHR documentation, what additional information is needed?
2. What problems would you address and document?
3. What goals does the nurse discuss with the patient?
4. What specific interventions will meet these goals?
5. How would the nurse evaluate if the goals were met?
6. According to Roy's theory, how is the client coping?
7. How does coping affect his present state?

Food for Thought

Integrating Lifelong Learning Into Nursing Practice

My earliest childhood memory took place when I was 4 years old. I remember having many earaches and sore throats as a young child. I know my parents were concerned because both my grandmother and mother had experienced hearing loss and wore hearing aids. One early morning, in the middle of a typical week, I noticed that my dad had stayed home from work. Both parents told me that we were "going to the library." I always loved going to the library; however, we passed right by the red brick library in the car.

We came upon another large red brick building that I recognized as my pediatrician's office. I remember being ushered into an examining room and held down while someone placed a cone over my face. The smell coming from that cone was indescribably bad. Later on in life, I learned that ether was used as an anesthetic for surgery in the 1950s.

I recall waking up in a "ward," full of crying, screaming kids. There had to be at least 20 kids in that room. My 4-year-old self reasoned: "Well, everyone else is screaming.... I guess I should too." I howled my head off. I later learned in nursing school that this activity is extremely dangerous post-tonsillectomy, as it could lead to hemorrhaging. My discharge to home came none too soon. My parents rescued me from the din, scooped me up and put me in the car, accompanied by a huge emesis basin. Once home, I can still remember the blood in that basin. Eventually, the bleeding stopped, and I recovered. Luckily, my sore throats and earaches disappeared too. My memories of this experience included unlimited Jello and the attention from everyone.

Years later, working as a pediatric nurse, equipped with the lifelong learning principles of informed, current knowledge, anticipatory guidance, and patient education ingrained in my head, I cared for tonsillectomy and adenoidectomy (T&A) patients. We educated parents during the perioperative period regarding what to expect for their children, letting the kids "sleep off the anesthesia," medicating them for pain, offering ice chips in the immediate post-op period, then adding popsicles and ice cream. I learned that these important measures would prevent the kids' crying for long periods of time. Along with a nursing degree, my earliest childhood memory, still vivid today, has served me well as a nurse.

References

Alligood, M. (2022). *Nursing theorists and their work* (10th ed.). Elsevier.

Anton, N., Hornbeck, T., Modlin, S., Haque, M., Crites, M., & Yu, D. (2021). Identifying factors that nurses consider in the decision-making process related to patient care during the COVID-19 pandemic. *PLoSOne,16*(7), e0254077. https://doi.org/10.1371/journal.pone.0254077

Benner, P., & Tanner, C. (1987). Clinical judgment: How expert nurses use intuition. *American Journal of Nursing, 87*(1), 23–31.

Ghanbari-Afra, L., Adib-Hajbaghery, M., & Dianati, M. (2022). Human caring: A concept analysis. *Journal of Caring Science, 2022*(4). https://doi.org/10.34172/jcs.2022.21

Hassani, P., Abdi, A., & Jalali, R. (2016). State of science, "intuition in nursing practice": A systematic review study.*Journal of Clinical and Diagnostic Research, 10*(2), JE07JE11. https://doi.org/10.7860/JCDR/2016/17385.7260

Melin-Johansson, C., Palmqvist, R., & Rönnberg, L. (2017). Clinical intuition in the nursing process and decision-making-A mixed-studies review. *Journal of Clinical Nursing*, *26*(23–24), 3936–3949. https://doi.org/10.1111/jocn.13814

Mlambo, M., Silén, C., & McGrath, C. (2021). Lifelong learning and nurses' continuing professional development: A metasynthesis of the literature. *BMC Nursing, 20(*62). https://doi.org/10.1186/s12912-021-00579-2

Montano, A.-R. (2021). Neuman systems model with nurse-led interprofessional collaborative practice. *Nursing Science Quarterly, 234*(1), 45–53.

Roy, C. (2009). *The Roy adaptation model* (3rd ed.). Pearson.

Swanson, K. M. (1991). Empirical development of a middle range theory of caring. *Nursing Research, 40(3)*, 161–165.

Turan, N., Özdemir, A. G., & Ozsaban, A. (2019). Intuition and emotional intelligence: A study in nursing students. *Cogent Psychology, 6*(1),1633077.

Figure Credits

Fig. 7.1: Angelo Gonzalo, https://nurseslabs.com/betty-neuman-systems-model-nursing-theory/. Copyright © 2024 by Nurseslabs.

Fig. 7.2: Adapted from Kristen M. Swanson, "Empirical Development Of a Middle Range Theory of Caring," *Nursing Research*, vol. 40, no. 3, https://journals.lww.com/nursingresearchonline/abstract/1991/05000/empirical_development_of_a_middle_range_theory_of.8.aspx. Copyright © 1991 by Wolters Kluwer Health.

■ CHAPTER 8

Resilience

The greatest glory in living lies not in never falling, but in rising every time we fall.

—Nelson Mandela

Introduction

Chapter 8 integrates theory, personal narratives, and actionable guidance to support nurses' resilience, presented through their stories of professional and personal challenges faced and strategies employed during the COVID-19 pandemic. Theories of Peplau and Kolcaba support caring and emotional processing, holistic approaches to care encouraging self-awareness, diversity appreciation, and career alignment. Readers are introduced to the challenges of "staying grounded" during traumatic events that impact nurses' personal and professional lives.

Han et al. (2023) define resilience as the capacity to "recover, adapt, and stay engaged" in the face of critical events in the workplace. Valued as an early indicator of potential burnout, resilience involves "decompression," nurses' ability to recover emotionally from work-related stress, and "activation," nurses' capacity to stay involved, inspired, and determined while encountering workplace challenges.

For health care organizations, staff resilience is important in fostering job satisfaction and retention, as well as in achieving quality care and outcomes for patients. Along with early and vigilant identification of factors threatening nurses' ability to recover during crisis, leadership strategies to recognize and facilitate those actions that maintain nurses' resilience are essential in administrators' commitment to the support of the work force.

Critical Incident One

Collaboration and Resiliency in a Pandemic

Every member of the health care industry was directly or indirectly affected by the COVID-19 virus and its consequences. Nurses played a significant and critical role in this struggle. Comprising more than 50% of providers, nurses faced overwhelming conditions to care for their patients. Whether pregnant, breastfeeding, elderly, students, or high-risk comorbid patients themselves, nurses placed their patients before their own families, and before their own health. The following critical incidents are just two examples of the many heroic acts of nurses working on the front lines of the COVID-19 pandemic.

> *I never thought that I'd be on the front lines of a pandemic in my first year as a nurse. This pandemic has rattled many of us in ways we have never experienced before. It's brought a lot of fear and uncertainty. I work in acute care on a res-*

piratory unit and treat many COVID-19 patients. Despite some of the challenges that I've faced (i.e., lack of PPE), I am heartened by the amazing support of my colleagues. Whenever I'm in a patient's room, with full protective equipment on, I can always count on my colleagues to gather the supplies I need. This pandemic has really shown me the importance of teamwork. It has allowed me to overcome many obstacles. It has also reminded me of the reason I decided to pursue a career in the medical field. My will to help people and care for them drives me through this crisis.

This nurse credits both her colleagues for their collaborative support and the nursing theorist Hildegard Peplau (1952) for her inspiration in guiding and educating patients during this tumultuous time:

Peplau maintains that the nurse makes a substantial difference in what each patient will learn while receiving nursing care. Peplau's theory explains roles and methods in nursing as an interpersonal process. Specifically meaningful to me is the identification phase, which relates to exploring the needs of the patient and the importance of the nurse assisting patients with their feelings while sustaining a positive environment. The COVID-19 pandemic is one that has created such fear, not only with our patients but also with health care workers. It is imperative to maintain a positive environment at all times for the health and wellness for all involved. Peplau's framework for therapeutic behavior of nurses aided in identifying ways to decrease anxiety and stress in patients. I was unaware of the impact making the decision I did was going to have on my nursing practice, but it has. I am focused. I am determined. I am positive in knowing we will get through this.

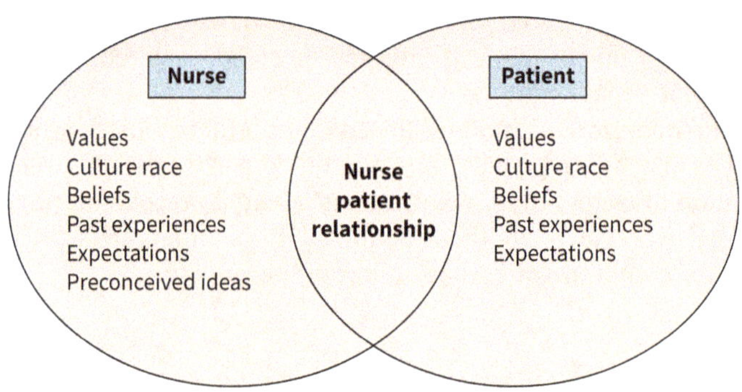

Figure 8.1 Peplau's Interpersonal Relations Theory

Nursing theorists and their theories frequently intersected during the COVID-19 pandemic: Orem, offering self-care with health education in virus prevention, home isolation with worsening of COVID-19; Nightingale, symbolizing environmental sanitation, ventilation, personal and domestic cleaning and the surrounding areas; Peplau, identifying therapeutic behaviors of nurses to decrease anxiety and stress in patients; Roy, mobilizing perceptions of focal stimuli, with the recognition of COVID symptoms, the contextual stimuli of comorbidities, and with residual stimuli, identifying the impact of work stress with factors such as high viral transmission and the scarcity of personal protective equipment (PPE).

This impressive base of nursing theories, frameworks, and models characterizes nursing from other professions (Almeida et al., 2020; Victor, 2022). While nurses may not always stop and reflect on their personal nursing theory philosophies, they incorporate nursing theories in their practice, particularly in tough times. This was made readily apparent in nurses' dedication to their patients during the COVID-19 crisis.

Nurses have been shown to persevere in maintaining the human connection that their patients need to heal, despite the challenges and barriers presented. For example, during their work on the front lines of the COVID-19 pandemic, nurses were not able to "shelter in place" with their own families. They did not have the luxury of maintaining a distance of 6 feet from extremely sick people. The public relied on their courage and sacrifices when facing daunting challenges each shift. Nurses honored their commitment to the profession by returning each day to face the same unknown, to repeat the same actions.

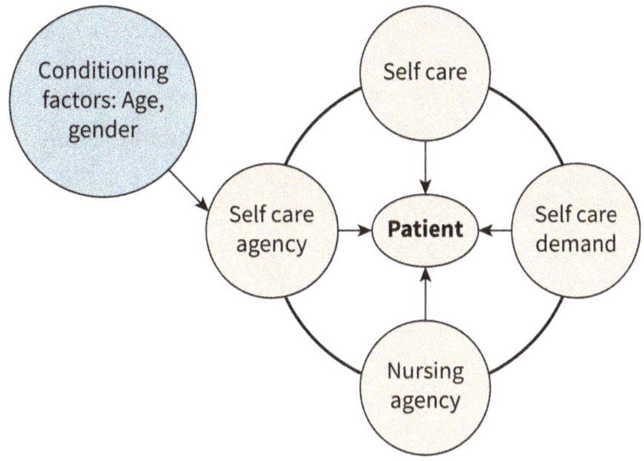

Figure 8.2 Orem's Self-Care Deficit Theory

Nurses demonstrate the remarkable ability to support others during their own individual periods of vulnerability. To risk peril in their work so that others may stay safe at home demands an uncommon degree of selflessness and bravery. To this day, years after the COVID-19 pandemic, a truly unparalleled time of fear and uncertainty, we thank these noble heroes for the miracles they continue to achieve.

Critical Incident Two

Advocacy, Ethics, and Resiliency

I will never forget the day that our dementia floor was transformed to a COVID-19 unit. Somehow, I knew it would happen, as my unit had already lost nearly half our residents to the virus, and other long-term care facilities were doing the same thing. Nevertheless, during a time when nothing was certain, resources were scarce, and people were scared, we had to carry on in a world where the rules seemed to change by the hour.

Of all the events that occurred, one case of procedural variation stuck with me. A family was allowed in for a compassionate visit as their loved one was passing. They had already agreed to care and comfort measures, and all end-of-life medication was on board. When the daughter, who also was the patient's HCP (health care proxy) arrived, she decided she wanted to send her mother to the hospital, hoping that they could treat her. After explaining the possible outcomes of a hospital transfer and the care that we provide, the HCP still insisted on sending her. Once the EMT arrived, they informed the daughter that they were no longer taking patients with a DNR order, and given the dementia diagnosis plus other comorbidities, the hospital most likely would not elect to treat her mother.

After the EMTs left, I attempted to comfort the daughter by explaining that her mother is not in any distress, and the staff has taken care of her for so long that the continuity is often just as important. Although she agreed that we had always treated her mom as family, she felt that she needed to give her mother one last chance. The daughter changed her mother's code status to a full code and called for her own emergency transport to a hospital where her sister was employed. The patient expired 2 days later.

The incident impacted me directly as I was the primary nurse in care of the patient. Two issues stuck out during situation. First, one of the EMTs informed me (outside of the room) that they were not taking any patients that were near death, and that even if we changed her code status, they would most likely still refuse to transport her. Second, it bothered me that the patient who had been with us for so long (and frequently only responded well with staff members that she recognized) had to endure an ambulance ride to an unfamiliar place and die with unfamiliar staff in a hospital that was not allowing family visits at all. Although the power was out of my hands, I lost sleep over the incident. I have a different compassion for end-of-life care philosophy as a result of this event. In my practice, now that resources are available again, I really push for hospice and social work to support families in benefit of patients' needs.

Vulnerable populations include those requiring utmost care, ancillary considerations, and augmented protections (Shivayogi, 2013). Those with the inability to make informed choices are included in the list. Because my patient had a diagnosis of dementia, she is considered unable to make informed decisions and therefore vulnerable. Part of a nurse's job is to identify and protect those at risk. Unfortunately, even after educating the family, the HCP had the ultimate decision.

The comfort theory by Katherine Kolcaba (2020) depicts comfort in three forms including relief, ease, and transcendence in relation to physical psychospiritual, environmental, and sociocultural aspects. Relief occurs when a specific comfort need is met, such as pain. Ease is the status of contentment and calmness. Transcendence is met when one can rise above challenges. The idea is that nurses assess the comfort needs of patients and families and implement interventions to meet those needs to enhance comfort and well-being. Included in the framework is achieving a peaceful death. Kolcaba and Bice (1997) define a peaceful death as death in which conflicts have been resolved, symptoms are well managed, and acceptance by the patient and family members allows for the patient to let go quietly and with dignity. The authors (Kolcaba & Bice, 1997) provide research and topics to help facilitate palliative care discussions with families of terminal patients. This theory may have impacted the critical incident that I described by providing additional resources and information for the family of the patient.

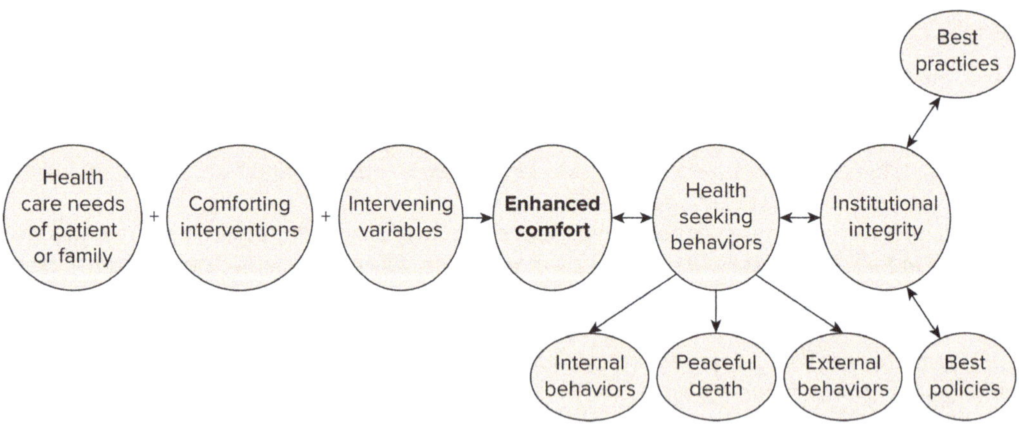

Figure 8.3 Conceptual Framework for Comfort Theory

Reflective Questions

1. What strategies should be included in developing self-care and resilience?
2. What signs of burnout might you identify in yourself and/or others?
3. What strategies might you devise to foster a supportive and resilient culture in the workplace?

4. Develop your own personal self-care and resilience plan. What would it look like?

Scenario

Combating Burnout: Self-Care and Resiliency

For 3 years, "Ava" has been a dedicated registered nurse, working full-time nights (11 p.m.–7 a.m.) in a long-term care facility since her graduation from nursing school. For the past three months, however, she has been feeling "off." She has always loved her work and has consistently received positive employee evaluations. She feels drained, disinterested and emotionally exhausted and has recently begun to dread going to work. During the past year, three nursing home residents Ava has been close to have passed away. Additionally, there has been a change in the organization's administration and a rise in staff turnover, sick calls, and staff shortages. Ava's supervisor, Leonard, recognizes that she might be exhibiting signs of burnout. He schedules a meeting to share his concerns with Ava and asks how he might help.

Setting Achievable Goals and Tracking Progress

In developing Ava's "Resiliency Plan" (with Ava), Leonard includes Ava's:

- Self-care ability
- Emotional well-being
- Physical well-being
- Exercise routine
- Workload (night shift/circadian rhythm)
- Sleep patterns
- Nutritional status
- Socialization/recreation
- Mentoring/peer support
- Professional support systems
- Future career plans

Other aspects to consider?
Outcomes: Measurable, realistic, attainable within a specific time frame?
Evaluation: Consider the long-term sustainability of this plan.

Food for Thought

To the Future Generation of Nurses

To our grandchildren, born and unborn, who constantly inspire us to keep first things first.

—Stephen Covey

Below is a basic guide to help you navigate the unexpected, inevitable, challenging moments that come your way in life. Without having a crystal ball to predict the future, what I can do is to prepare you as I was prepared, as were my parents and grandparents, to help in your journey.

- **Cherish time**. Despite what you may think and depending how old you are when you read this, your time on the planet is brief, so make the most of it. The meaning of life is to give significance to our time here. Each one of us must decide what will be our purpose, which depends on one's perspective. For me, a purposeful life includes caring for people, inspiring, learning, and helping. Having chosen a career in nursing, and seeing how fleeting life is, I have always been aware of the importance of making each day count.
- **Appreciate diversity**. As crazy as they make you (and you them), I would encourage all generations and all populations to spend more time together. I know it is important to pass on wisdom for the future; however, it is just as important to learn from the living, right now. Too, each generation should encourage them and support one another. My grandmother always advised "take the time to smell the roses." My parents taught me to have a path in life. My mentors helped me to learn from my mistakes and to never give up. Patients taught me about their culture. These life experiences contributed to finding daily meaning in life and to understand the perspectives of others.
- **Find your niche.** Do not stay in a job where you are unhappy. Dreading each day as you enter the workplace is self-destructive and energy-sapping. If it is making you anxious, sick, and sleepless, it is time to leave. If you feel you cannot contribute to this position or organization, you have not failed; you have succeeded by recognizing that this job does not give you the opportunity to learn, grow, and contribute. If you can muster the self-confidence and courage to move on to an environment where you seek appreciation and acceptance and where you can make a difference, it will happen. Experience teaches us to ask questions when interviewing for a new position. Have faith in the knowledge that nursing offers many opportunities and pathways. Rest assured that it won't be long before you find your place.
- **Cherish learning**. Make the most of your nursing education. Nursing school was an important wake-up call. It was by far one of the best decisions I have made in my life. To be a participant in some of the most intimate moments in a person's life is an honor and a privilege. Nursing also offers a flexible schedule where one can raise a family, work in all areas of the profession, experience lifelong learning, and have an opportunity each day to make a difference. It also provided a wake-up call that life is fleeting. As 18-year-old nursing students in Anatomy and Physiology class, we were shown the shocking and grim image differences between the lungs of smokers and nonsmokers. At the same time, my 82-year-old grandfather was suffering from emphysema. Considering his history (smoking since the age of nine, a lifelong housepainter, and a veteran "gassed" in WWI), this made me realize how casually we regard the simple act of breathing. Grandpa could not walk to the kitchen from the living room without choking and coughing. He spent the last years of his life homebound, tethered to an oxygen tank. Learning happens everywhere, every day. I never picked up a cigarette.
- **Expect lifelong learning**. Never stop learning. There is so much to know! Life is a complex trail of learning experiences, all merging to tell many stories. It is not the end goal or outcome of life that gives life meaning but rather the "ride" itself. Be in the moment. Do not waste a minute on events over which you have no control: dwelling on the past; the weather, other peoples' lives, the "what ifs," the future; mistakes we have made in the past. Learn from the experience and move forward.
- **Practice transparency**. There can be no singular meaning of life to stand for us all, or even any one of us. Take the time to listen to others and gain an understanding of their perspective. New and different revelations about life are not easy to accept. Do not let the things you disagree with stop you from investigating further. Life is a balance of duties and enjoyment. Only in this way can we satisfy both ourselves and the people

around us. Living our lives for the people around us and ourselves are interconnected. Seeing the people around us happy should bring us joy.

- **Be grateful.** My best advice to future nurses is, every so often, to take the time to treasure what you have. I am not talking about the "stuff" we accumulate but appreciating the world and the people around us. Gratitude means dare to ask questions, walk in the shoes of others, respect the wisdom of the ages, and never hesitate to thank others for their help. From our collective experience in the time of the COVID-19 pandemic, I would hope that this experience has taught us to better appreciate and to impress upon others the need to "smell the roses."
- **Leave a legacy**. Live with purpose. Find meaning to fulfill or satisfy your needs. Purpose is something to live for and something to look forward to in life. Find your passion. One's happiness lies in having things to look forward to in life and to wake up the next morning to enjoy the new day. Savor the simple things in a life of rushing: watching the bird, planting a garden from seeds, reading for pleasure, appreciating the change of seasons, sleeping, and living in the moment. In the words of Stephen Covey, "No one on their death bed wished they had spent more time at the office." Carpe diem.

References

Almeida, I. J. S., Lúcio, P. D. S., Nascimento, M. F. D., & Coura, A. S. (2020). Coronavirus pandemic in light of nursing theories. *Revista brasileira de enfermagem*, *73*(suppl 2), e20200538. https://doi.org/10.1590/0034-7167-2020-0538

Covey, S. R., & Collins, J.C.L. (2013). *The 7 habits of highly effective people: Powerful lessons in personal change* (25th anniv. ed.). Simon & Schuster.

Covey, S. R., Merrill, A. R., & Merrill, R. R. (1994). *First things first: To live, to love, to learn, to leave a legacy.* Simon & Schuster.

Han, P., Duan, X., Jiang, J., Zeng, L., Zhang, P., & Zhao, S. (2023). Experience in the development of nurses' personal resilience: A meta-synthesis. *Nursing Open*, *10*(5), 2780–2792. https://doi.org/10.1002/nop2.1556

Kolcaba, K. (2020). *Comfort theory.* Current Nursing. Retrieved November 29, 2021, from https://www.currentnursing.com/nursing_theory/comfort_theory_Kathy_Kolcaba.html

Kolcaba, K., & Bice, A. (1997). *End of life and palliative care: The comfort line*. Comfort Line. Retrieved November 30, 2021, from https://www.thecomfortline.com/end-of-life-care

Orem D. (2001). *Nursing: Concepts of practice* (5th ed.). Mosby.

Peplau, H. E. (1952). *Interpersonal relations in nursing: A conceptual frame of reference for psychodynamic nursing*. Putnam.

Shivayogi, P. (2013). Vulnerable populations and methods for their safeguard. *Perspectives in Clinical Research*, *4*(1), 53. https://doi.org/10.4103/2229-3485.106389

Victor, R. M. H (2022). Being a nurse according to Jean Watson: The reason for being and doing. *Nursology*. https://nursology.net/2022/06/21/being-a-nurse-according-to-jean-watson-the-reason-for-being-and-doing/

Figure Credits

Fig. 8.1: Hildegard E. Peplau, *Interpersonal Relations in Nursing: A Conceptual Frame of Reference for Psychodynamic Nursing*. Copyright © 1952 by G.P. Putnam's Sons.

Fig. 8.2: Dorothea E. Orem, *Nursing: Concepts of Practice*. Copyright © 2001 by Elsevier B.V.

Fig. 8.3: Johan Earl Cu, "Concepts and Definitions," *Katharine Kolcaba: The Comfort Theory*, https://2013upoujohanearlman.wordpress.com/2013/06/27/conceptual-and-definitions/. Copyright © 2013 by University of the Philippines Open University.

PART III

3 Looking Ahead

■ CHAPTER 9

Growing Our Own

As a single footstep will not make a path on the earth, so a single thought will not make a pathway in the mind. To make a deep physical path, we walk again and again. To make a deep mental path, we must think over and over the kind of thoughts we wish to dominate our lives.

—Henry David Thoreau

Introduction

Healthcare is experiencing a profound change from converging elements that have significantly increased the demand for the skills, expertise, and experience of nurses. Challenges that can deter the delivery of quality nursing care to patients include staffing shortages, high patient-to-nurse ratios, and limited resources. These factors contribute to time constraints, missed care and increased stress for all care providers (Algoso et al., 2024).

The COVID-19 pandemic drew attention to the essential role of nurses, working on the front lines, caring for patients, administering vaccines, and providing critical support during times of crisis. Dedicated nurses returned daily to care for their patients, despite exposure to an extremely dangerous and contagious virus in the workplace. This crisis emphasized the significance of the nursing profession in acute, long-term, and community health care settings and highlighted the need for a "formidable" nursing workforce. Over time, the stress of the pandemic took a toll, with escalating rates of depression and anxiety among nurses (Brown et al., 2023).

Preceding the COVID-19 pandemic, many parts of the country, urban and rural, were witnessing a rising nursing shortage (Brown et al., 2023). The aging population of baby boomers with chronic illnesses and comorbidities increased the overall demand for health care services. Their complex needs placed a greater emphasis on prevention, coordination, and long-term health care services, all of which depended heavily on the education, experience, and skills and dedication of nurses (Algoso et al., 2024).

Nurses approaching retirement age were leaving the workforce due to exhaustion, compassion fatigue, and burnout, along with concerns that they (and their families) were overly exposed to the virus. When a hospital cannot maintain safe staffing levels, those remaining nurses carry an additional workload, perpetuating a cycle of staff turnover. Additionally, academic nursing programs were put on hold due to clinical delays and cancellations. Ultimately, the postponement of "feeder" programs resulted in fewer new nurses entering the field (Algoso et al., 2024; Brown et al., 2023).

Advances in medical technology require complex treatments and diagnostics, as well as skilled nursing professionals to operate and manage these technologies effectively. Also, a growing emphasis on patient-centered care requires nurses to engage more actively in patient education, advocacy, and coordination of care across various health care providers and settings. Telemedicine and digital health solutions are also becoming integral components of health care delivery, expanding the scope of nursing practice to include remote patient monitoring and virtual consultations. With technology comes expectations of advanced skills for nurses (Algoso et al., 2024).

From this crisis there is good news on the horizon. The fallout from the pandemic was demonstrated in the public's gratitude and enthusiastic appreciation for nurses. The COVID-19 crisis highlighted the urgent issues in nursing, including caregiver burnout, a lack of mental health support, and challenging working conditions. Many organizations provide counseling services, peer support groups, workplace safety initiatives, and resilience training, along with endeavors to improve staff access to professional development opportunities and career advancement. A culture of leadership, action, and support is taking root, with mentorship programs emerging in many workplaces to help nurses thrive. Efforts continue in addressing ongoing challenges of reducing mandatory overtime hours, ensuring healthy staffing levels, and promoting a healthy work-life balance.

In strategizing for success to resolve the multiple challenges facing the nursing profession today, it is imperative to start at the top. Nursing leaders are needed to troubleshoot and support the goals of a collaborative effort of willing individuals, invested in turning things around. In the leadership role, it is the responsibility of the chief nursing officer (CNO) to enlist the skills of staff and interdisciplinary providers and to welcome the voices of community members. Public participation helps to spread community awareness of the day-to-day management of health care organizations, and how these challenges affecting health care providers trickle down to the public's use of health care systems. It is crucial that frontline nursing leaders be present and long-term members of the organization to help promote continual support, foster multidisciplinary collaboration among staff and community members, maintain a strong culture of problem-solvers, and invest in maintaining quality, longevity, and pride in their health care organizations.

The Nursing Shortage

There is a global shortage of six million nurses (National Council of State Boards of Nursing, 2021). U.S. hospital turnover rates within the first year of employment are at 31%, with 1-year rates being 27.7% and 19.2% at 2 years (NSI Nursing Solutions Inc, 2022). Continually losing new nurses is costly for organizations, which has prompted leaders to seek interventions for turnover and new retention strategies.

The rising shortage of nurses is a present and pressing concern (Lee, 2024; Tamata & Mohammadnezhad, 2023). Contributing factors to this shortage are many: the nursing educatorshortage; the retirement of an aging workforce; a growing demand for health care services from an aging population; workplace violence, stress, and burnout; and increased pressure to integrate and master advanced technology into practice (American Association of Colleges of Nursing [AACN], 2024).

Data from the U.S. Bureau of Labor Statistics cites the need for 275,000 additional nurses by 2030 to meet the growing needs for nurses to replace retiring clinicians and educators. The current stress on health care systems is apparent, intensified by the health care needs of an aging baby boomer population and the long-term effects of the COVID-19 pandemic. Other contributing factors point to nurses exiting the workplace due to burnout, high nurse to patient staffing ratios, inadequate institutional support, and lack of a work-life balance (Haddad et al., 2023).

As Americans age, demand for healthcare continues to increase at an exceptional rate. The U.S. Census Bureau reports that by 2030, 73 million baby boomers will reach age 65 years of age or older. We are now living longer than our predecessors. This substantial segment of the population will require additional health services, placing a significant strain on existing and burdened health care resources (U.S. Census, Bureau 2019).

The Nursing Shortage: Growing Our Own

Confronting the nursing shortage requires schools and health care providers to recruit new nurses and support working conditions that reduce turnover. Federal and state governments, career and health advocacy organizations have developed programs to attract and retain nurses. One example is the Nursing Education Loan Repayment program, which repays up to 85% of educational loans for nurses who work in qualifying facilities in areas with critical nursing shortages (Health Resources and Services Administration, 2026).

With healthcare becoming more complex, organizations are finding an increasing need to create "transition to practice" (TTP) courses (Lee, 2024). Such programs aid in building novice nurses' confidence in practice. For new graduate registered nurses (NGRNs), TTP utilizes active learning to support progression from prelicensure nursing education into licensed practice.

More hospitals are recognizing the importance of TTP programs on clinical skill development, practice readiness, and socialization of their NGRNs. Rush et al. (2019) found that providing NGRNs with evidence-based, standardized, TTP programs decreased turnover and increased retention. TTP programs that incorporate targeted classroom education, computer-based learning, clinical precepted time, and mentoring offer NGRNs optimal learning experiences.

For those contemplating a career in nursing, the following resources are offered:

- **The Career Pipeline**. Used to attract and inspire young people to consider nursing as a career, the pipeline partners high schools with universities and colleges in venues such as nursing career fairs, shadowing programs, and scholarships. These initiatives introduce students to the health care field and the wide array of areas in the discipline to explore. Beyond financial incentives, perks such as tuition reimbursement, student loan forgiveness, and flexible scheduling can help reduce the fear often associated with applying to college (Smiley et al., 2023).
- **Accessing Social Media.** An efficient and effective online recruitment strategy introducing potential nursing students to a particular program. Easily accessed on the college/university website, this resource efficiently summarizes information, showcasing a nursing program's curriculum, clinical setting locations, program success rates (NCLEX scores) career outcomes, and student testimonials, as well as emphasizing professional development opportunities, extracurricular activities, and support networks available to students.
- **Open Houses**. In this setting, nursing faculty and administration collaborate to welcome prospective students and their families to the campus, to showcase their program. The event is usually offered at specific times during the school year, often on the weekends. In a typical open house agenda and setting, nursing faculty present a general overview of the program, describe the curriculum, and provide sufficient time at the end of the day to answer individual questions. Clinical nursing instructors also volunteer to participate at open house. Employed at local clinical agencies and health care facilities, they are the "bridge" between academia and clinical placement.

Group tours of the campus take visitors through the dining hall and student housing. Current nursing students navigate visitors through the nursing department and learning laboratory, where they can view a simulation demonstration, followed by their attendance at a panel discussion (led by sophomore, junior, and senior nursing students) with a Q&A session centering around the nursing student experience. Visitors then return to the original meeting location to meet up with nursing faculty to answer any additional questions.

Feedback from open houses is consistently positive. Open house evaluations, in this author's experience, have shown that attendees enjoy the positive energy of the presentation, the ability to ask questions, a well-organized, efficient itinerary, and the chance to meet and talk one on one with faculty, staff and students.

For educators and administrators, campus visits provide the opportunity to highlight and showcase their education institution and their individual programs. In many settings, representatives from departments such as admissions,housing, financial aid, health and counseling, and tutoring services are present during open house to describe their programs and to field questions. Faculty, staff, and administration present evidence of the high percentage of students who graduate, obtain certifications, and secure jobs in their field of study. Presenters cite examples of their alumni's career paths, emphasizing the diverse opportunities available. They take pride in announcing any national rankings, accreditations, or awards the program has received. They model a welcoming environment for students from all backgrounds and highlight those resources to help students succeed.

The Nursing Faculty Shortage

According to the American Association of Colleges of Nursing's (AACN) 2023–2024 report, the average ages of doctorally prepared nurse faculty holding the ranks of professor, associate professor, and assistant professor were 61.2, 55.6, and 49.6 years, respectively (Rosseter, 2024). For master's-degree-prepared nurse faculty, the average ages for professors, associate professors, and assistant professors were 55.0, 54.7, and 47.5 years, respectively. Within the next decade, many of these nurses will retire, leaving gaps in the workplace and the potential for this population to fill educator vacancies. Maintaining a steady supply of nurses in the educator pipeline for future employment into academic positions requires continual exploration of resources for training and education (Antig et al., 2024).

The present scarcity of nursing faculty is seriously hindering admissions to nursing programs. As reported by the AACN (2023) in their "Nursing Workforce Fact Sheet," on enrollment and graduations in baccalaureate and graduate nursing programs, nursing schools turned away over 65,000 qualified applicants. This was largely due to the severe lack of faculty available to mentor the next generation of nurses. In 2023, AACN cited that 5,491 qualified master's and 4,461 doctoral applicants were turned away from these educational programs. Reasons given were shortage of advanced practice nursing faculty, preceptors, and clinical education sites (Rosseter, 2024).

Complicating this situation is the increasing number of nurse educators who are approaching retirement age, leading to a rapid decline in this workforce population. Furthermore, competition for faculty from clinical and private-sector employers, offering better pay and working conditions, attracts qualified educators away from traditional nursing programs. Additional research reports that doctoral programs are not producing qualified educators quickly enough to replace those leaving the field. As a result, the educator shortage is only expected to increase (Rosseter, 2024).

The Nursing Faculty Shortage: Reversing the Trend Through Mentoring

Mentoring is a way of conveying knowledge, using traditional wisdom, and employing the experiences of established colleagues, Historically, this concept of mentoring is a well-known narrative. In Greek mythology, Athena, the goddess of wisdom, mentored several Greek leaders during the Trojan War, characterized in Homer's *Iliad* (Homer, 1961).

According to many veteran educators, their success is attributed to guidance by experts in the field. For them, mentoring was a protective "buddy system." This informal "passing of the torch" from veteran to fledgling educator helped the novice "gain passage" to their experience, expertise, and wisdom (Chichester, 2009).

Both developmental and nursing theories support nurse mentoring as an opportunity for creating a professional legacy. Psychologist and psychoanalyst Erik Erikson (1950) described eight psychosocial stages of development. In his model, the tasks attributed to the middle years from 25–64 are to produce and nurture the next generation. This model is also applicable to experienced nurse mentors who seek to help mentees through socialization and by offering encouragement and support.

Mentors provide more than just the "how to" aspects of the job. Successful mentoring relationships are long term, develop between individuals with similar interests, and have mutual benefits for participants (Thorpe & Kalischuk, 2003). The National Leauge for Nursing (NLN, 2006b) position statement speaks to such an approach, involving mentoring across the career continuum, where mentoring is a belief of the community and where faculty and administrators are well-informed about benefits, attributes, and practices of effective mentoring relationships. Being a part of a mutually respected community of colleagues is confirmation of the collegiality and community involvement in mentoring. Experiencing these considerate exchanges is a component of academic work vital to all faulty members in higher education

In their research regarding theoretical underpinnings of technology-based interactive instruction, Khalid et al. (2024) credit technology with providing the tools to make communication successful and affording opportunities to develop innovative strategies for mentoring. Mentors and protégés can connect using various approaches such as electronic mail, video, and teleconferencing. The key to making this work is having a plan for regular and meaningful contact.

Before attending Project LEAD, a training program for minority educators in special education and educational leadership, Johnson (2007) believed mentoring was limited to neophyte nurses. After the program, she recognized the significance of having a mentor who understood her strengths and weaknesses and provided regular guidance. For Johnson, the Project LEAD experience exposed her to different leadership styles and demonstrated the need for mentorship on a regular basis. Johnson's mentor eased her transition from department chair to faculty member, where she was able to employ her newly acquired management skills to establish networks with community leaders (Johnson, 2007).

Horton (2003) described the importance of mentoring early on in a student's professional career. She included the characteristics of an expert educator as one who is an effective mentor to faculty members. Horton advised senior faculty to recruit and mentor promising students who desire growth and envision a career commitment, in order to retain them as future educators.

Thorpe and Kalischuk (2003) described the use of the collegial mentoring model. In this format, mentoring is a friendship-based, reciprocal association that affords sincere and open communication over an extended period of time, resulting in a positive outcome for both individuals. The authors view this model as a window of opportunity for recreating the nursing profession, enhancing the evolution of nursing, and helping to build a strong professional culture among nurse educators.

Patricia Benner's theoretical framework of "novice to expert" is another example of a mentoring model where novice nurse educators benefit from the knowledge and wisdom of a "proficient" or "expert" nurse educator as mentor. Role change from clinician to educator is a stressful and daunting venture. In her *novice to expert* model, Benner (2001) states that in the acquisition of a skill, an individual passes through five levels of proficiency: *novice, advanced beginner, competent, proficient, and expert*. The Benner model, which aids in the transition through nurses' developmental stages, can be applied to the progression of novice to expert nurse educators. In stage one, the*novice* nurse educator may be the nurse clinician who has recently begun a career in academia. Benner states that any individual entering into a new setting with no previous experience is at the novice level of performance, with different goals, expectations, and roles.

According to Benner's description at each stage, there is considerable difference between a *competent* and *expert* practitioner. The *competent* practitioner has 2 to 3 years of experience in the same setting, engages in conscious and purposeful planning, and uses an analytic framework. In comparison, the*expert* has practiced for six or more years in the same setting and does not rely on rules and analytic frameworks.

Barker (2006) describes role attainment as consisting of several stages, all of which eventually leads to excellence. The protégée, in this instance, the novice nurse educator, is significantly reliant on an adviser, or mentor. With support and experience over time, the protégé gains more autonomy and knowledge; eventually, the protégé becomes the mentor.

Academic preparation and clinical ability do not always provide novice nurse educators with a full awareness of the faculty position. With time, encouragement, and practice, novices should be able to practice and refine skills, scaffolding learning experiences toward competency in the educator role, eventually gaining proficient and expert nurse educator status. Scaffold learning begins with assistance by mentors to the self-learning of the mentee, toward the eventual goal of internalization. This higher-order learning emerges from contact with those who have more knowledge than the learner (Sanders & Welk, 2005).

Mentoring in nursing education is a professional conduit for transferring knowledge, skills, behaviors, and principles to a less experienced "mentee" (NLN, 2006c). In this setting, mentors have the opportunity to significantly influence the professional growth and development of a mentee. The work of the mentor is to lay the foundation for the future of nursing.

Many novice nurse educators enter academia from clinical practice, staff education, or part-time clinical teaching assignments. Once employed, they are challenged with navigating through unknown waters, including lecture and test construction, curriculum revision, committee assignments, and solving complex student issues. For the novice, guidance from an invested mentor helps to translate and make sense of the nurse educator role.

Mentors transfer their experience and knowledge to guide the mentee's personal and career development. Mentors are visionaries. They have expertise in networking and leadership skills, believe in the abilities of the mentee and advocate for their success.

In the role of the novice nurse educator, the mentee integrates an inspiration to learn with a readiness to accept and act on constructive feedback. The mentee is self-directed and has the capability and willingness to identify individual career goals. The mentee looks to the experienced nurse educator for steady, thoughtful, and consistent direction. A structured mentoring program can lead to a collegial and attentive association between mentor and mentee, fostering personal and professional growth.

Learning is an empowering and significant human experience. The opportunity to communicate knowledge through teaching is one of the most important undertakings we must accomplish as nursing educators. Excellence in teaching stems from the desire to learn and from the desire to communicate this information to others. Given the appropriate consideration and setting, learning is a sound investment for the future (National League for Nursing, 2006a).

Benefits of a Mentoring Program

For the mentee

- Gaining knowledge about policies, job responsibilities, and culture of the organization
- Receiving emotional support to ease many concerns and anxieties
- Improving teaching performance and promoting student learning
- Engaging in professional growth activities that enhance knowledge of effective strategies
- Systematically building on successful educational practice
- Choosing to remain in the teaching profession

For the mentor

- Becoming a more reflective practitioner
- Recognizing the challenges of systemic change
- Securing the ability to transfer the knowledge and skills in effective practice
- Communicating enthusiasm and motivation for teaching
- Advancing in leadership skills
- Growing professionally (of self and others)

For administration

- Supporting efforts to improve the quality and effectiveness of faculty education
- Building collaboration within the school that encourages collegial problem-solving
- Promoting positive professional growth
- Assisting in the identification and resolution of problems faced by novice nurse educators

For the educational institution

- Retaining quality nurse educators who understand the organizational culture
- Identifying and assisting new teachers in resolving problems
- Creating teacher professional training through learning communities
- Demonstrating best practices for support and achievement of nursing faculty and students

The Nurse Educator in Academia

Understanding the lived experience of nursing faculty members provides insight for administrators, students, and clinicians into what it is truly like to live this role. Education in this role needs to include what nurse educators do, the voices of experienced nurses considering a career in academia, the preparation of educators, and the ways in which they are welcomed into the educational community. Being a nurse educator necessitates working in surroundings where teaching is appreciated, respected, and supported. The educational setting must be flexible in how it integrates individual educators' contributions of skill and expertise to the overall teaching effort.

Research purports that values developed by students throughout their education may be affected in different degrees by the nurse educators to whom the student is exposed. Haigh and Johnson (2007) conducted an interview of nurse educators from 19 different countries. Educators reported high regard for the values of honesty and intellectualism, while maintaining a more cautious, although still positive, attitude toward altruism in healthcare. The study illustrates the importance of educators' strengths related to values and attitudes. Honesty, altruism, and intellectualism are viewed as significant strengths of nurse educators.

Dempsey (2007) examined the experiences of clinical nurses in Ireland who transitioned to the role of nurse lecturer. Themes emerging from the study included role stressors, educational preparation, and the availability of support systems.

In a study of novice nursing faculty conducted by Silas and Kleiner (2001), findings revealed that educators' expectations were contrary to what actually took place, and that novice educators were unprepared both educationally and experientially for the multiple role expectations. Educators stated that they were unfamiliar with the language, culture, and practices of the new role, and the workload was much greater than they expected.

Assistant professors from the University of North Carolina described innovative strategies to decrease stress for the new faculty challenges. Heavy workloads, adherence to the university's way of life, pressure to attain tenure status, increased emphasis on technological competence, and the need to maintain expertise in one's field all illustrated the importance of having a mentor. This study described a creative approach to enhance role success through the initiation of a personal and professional self-governing support group (Lewallen et al., 2003).

The Novice Nurse Educator: Orientation to the Faculty Role

Orientation to the role of faculty member should include provision of support, guidance, and resources from a designated mentor, whether it be seasoned faculty, the nursing department chair, the dean of nursing, or a mentoring team. Role development is enhanced through a detailed review and discussion of the job description, promotion and tenure, examination of the NLN's Core Competencies of Nurse Educators, and review of guidelines for clinical education experiences, as outlined by the particular state board of nursing. Ensuring that the new faculty member has access to electronic and/or hard copies of the program's latest self-study provides a comprehensive overview of the program, the institution and the "fit" of the new faculty member into the curriculum. Other documents that the novice faculty member must have access to include electronic and/or hard copies of the nursing student handbook, the college catalog, and both college employee and nursing faculty handbook. However, it is not enough to distribute these manuals and to expect that the novice will be able to digest, understand, and implement the guidelines flawlessly. They must be viewed as a supplement and not a replacement for carrying out a continuous, consistent, organized mentoring program and open dialogue for the novice nurse educator.

Preparation for the role of student adviser is an important expectation of all nurse faculty. Advising includes guiding students with course selection, progression policies, and preparing for the licensing examination. This complex role requires thorough individual mentoring. A working knowledge of all program options available to students is essential in order to advise students appropriately. An essential component of a comprehensive formal mentoring program must include sessions where the mentees observe the mentor in the advising process. Subsequently, the mentor will observe the mentee conducting an advising session, and faculty-student advising sessions will be discussed and critiqued.

Implications for Nursing Practice

As the nursing education faculty shortage drives efforts to attract larger numbers of nurses considering nursing education as a career, those individuals will undoubtedly experience stressors in their new roles. New faculty would benefit from the development of transition programs and support groups offering personal and professional rewards while facilitating success with the role change (Antig et al., 2024).

Feedback and support from a mentor, whether an individual or a team, allows the novice educator to better understand the daily responsibilities and expectations of the position. While an expert clinician, the novice educator may know very little about the overall curriculum, lesson planning, or test construction. In a mentoring relationship, the novice educator is able to better navigate the system. Focusing on these activities before any errors occur, the novice educator becomes more effective, assumes an increased comfort level, builds self-esteem as an educator, and ultimately stays in the role.

Reflective Questions

1. What aspects of the nursing profession do you find most interesting?
2. Do the critical incidents portrayed in this book help you to better understand what nurses do?
3. Identify qualities or strengths an individual should possess to consider a career in nursing.
4. Has reading about the challenges in the nursing profession affected your decision in any way?
5. What are your thoughts about the role mentors play?

Scenario

Success in the Mentoring Experience

During an assigned senior nursing student preceptorship during his last semester (12 weeks) in an entry level baccalaureate program, Arthur (the "mentee") was paired with veteran (14 years) registered nurse Leona (the "mentor") on a 40-bed medical-surgical hospital unit. Each week during their time together, mentor and mentee schedule one hour for "interviews." They chose this name as a symbol of collegiality when reflecting on each other's collective progress together during this collaborative preceptorship experience. As the following example illustrates, the typical interview dialogue encourages collaboration and professional growth for both participants. In this scenario, Arthur is initiating today's discussion:

> *Arthur:* ***What made you choose to be a mentor?***
>
> *Leona: The first year working as an RN was especially difficult. I started out on a medical-surgical unit. I felt overwhelmed most of the time. Luckily, I was "informally" mentored by experienced nurse, with years of experience. They encouraged me to seek them out for advice and guidance regarding my struggles during that first year out of nursing school. I recognized early on in my practice the need to "pay it forward"...to help new graduates "connect the dots" between academics and clinical practice. I have been a mentor on this unit for the past 7 years.*

Leona: ***Here's a question you probably were never asked. As a mentee, how would YOU define the role of the mentor?***

Arthur: I knew you would ask this question! So I made a list!

Sharing knowledge and life experiences

Offering encouragement and inspiration and enthusiasm for what you do

Listening when needed and providing guidance or advice when asked

Assisting the mentee to set goals*during the mentorship experience*

Fostering development of the mentee's leadership skills

Arthur: ***What advice would you give to nurses considering mentoring a new graduate?***

Leona: First and foremost, invest time in getting to know your mentee. Both individuals need to work together to decide the structure of your mentorship, examine the goals set forth by both the nursing program and the hospital organization's mission and vision? Are they realistic?

Leona: ***As a mentor, delivering constructive criticism can be challenging. From your perspective, how can feedback be best presented?***

Arthur: I think timing of the feedback and the actual delivery of the information are really important. We know that respect, compassion, active listening, and appropriate language on both ends are skills but in the heat of the moment, it sometimes triggers emotions. So it may be wise to let the feedback sit for a minute before responding. It's also good to hear positive comments…what's going well, along with those areas needing improvement.

Leona: I agree that the delivery should be straightforward and that active listening ensures that both parties are understanding the issues correctly. We can then move forward to work together for a resolution.

Arthur: I have to add that while mentors may be able to help their mentee find a solution to problems, the mentor can't totally fix everything. I think that letting the mentee know that you're available and willing to listen and brainstorm together really opens the door to communication and guides the mentee to critically think through the problem-solving process.

Arthur: ***I remember during "Communication" classes in Fundamentals of Nursing the importance of using the acronym WAIT—why am I talking—to help communicate effectively and reflect on what you're trying to articulate****. Is what I'm saying adding value to the conversation? Is what I'm saying repeating information already said during the conversation? Asking these questions helps constantly add value to a discussion and can help build a stronger mentor-mentee. When I get nervous, I tend to talk a lot, so this helped me to focus, especially useful when teaching patients in the clinical setting.*

Leona: So you just taught ME something I didn't know. Thanks for the tip!

Questions for Further Discussion

- From the previous brief discussion, what therapeutic communication techniques do you recognize that cultivate the mentoring relationship?
- How do missteps and failures help with critical thinking and problem-solving skills?
- Arthur recommends that during a constructive criticism "interview," the mentor include the strengths of the mentee. How does this foster investment in the mentee's success?
- What additional questions, comments or input might you contribute after reading this interview?
- From this mentoring experience, can you envision a future career in advanced practice in leadership or nursing education roles for Leona and Arthur? Why?

Food for Thought

Inspiration From the Past

As you contemplate your future career plans, take some encouragement from a former speech to nursing graduates at Montachusett Regional Vocational Technical School in 2018.

Honored guests, graduates, family, and friends,

Thank you for the honor and opportunity to address you all tonight. Among the highest honors that can be bestowed upon an individual is a nursing degree. It is an honor that I understand the value of now more than I would have at any other time in my career. I understand the value of what we all do as health care professionals. I have seen the differences that we can make. It won't be long before you'll begin to understand the value of what you do. Right now, you're just beginning your adventure. And it's going to be an adventure. The people and experiences you will encounter will be unpredictable and wonderful, fascinating, and frustrating, heart-wrenching and humbling.

You will remember this day as one of the most important days in your life. It is a time for you to look back and yet, at the same time, to look ahead at a world that awaits your valuable contributions. It is a time for heartfelt reflections as you think of family, friends, special times, personal study, and dedicated educators who helped lead you to this appointed hour of graduation. You no doubt have been encouraged and supported by those who unfailingly loved you, who cautiously guided you, and who thoughtfully advised you from the early years of your life to the person who sits before us today. The awareness you sensed that others strongly believed in you probably strengthened the belief that you had in yourself. So, here you are today at one of the greatest moments of your life, looking toward your future and, in a sense, toward the unknown.

Along the way, you will find your calling. In a speech at Harvard, Bono, lead singer of the band U2, challenged graduates to find "the hole in your hearts": Why are you here? Why do you have to listen? What have you given up to get here? What is your potential? Is missing the moment unacceptable to you? If so, this is where we find our lives' rhyme, our potential, our calling.

With the changes that are taking place in healthcare today, you will have more opportunities than anyone before you to find that calling. As tomorrow's nurses, you have the ability to accomplish so much! You have the skills to develop, use, and to challenge evidence. You know how to critically examine information and change it. It is up to you how you decide to use all of those skills to make a difference.

Making a difference means committing to and never losing track of the values and the mission to making our health care system more responsive, more effective, and more equitable in providing quality care. It is about being authentic and connected to your own values and those of the nursing profession, about having a voice and being vigilant in affecting fundamental changes in your practice setting.

Although we have made progress in healthcare, it is nothing compared to what we are experiencing in the information age, or what will take place over the next 100 years. We are expecting new and growing challenges with a greater percentage of the population approaching 70. Professionals now have better access to evidence-based information to help them, and their patients make better, more informed decisions about their health care options. Evidence on outcomes is readily available through the use of health information technology.

You are graduating at a time when the evolving face of healthcare requires a great deal of adaptability to change. You are the next generation of health care providers, and it is important for you to see yourselves as change agents who will impact the future of healthcare for years to come. Speak up for patient-centered care. Contribute as team members with other health professionals and be a vocal and important part of your teams. Each of us bears a responsibility for ensuring the health outcomes for the populations we serve.

Strive for lifelong learning connectedness, flexibility, respect, communication. Also, remember that even though you don't always hear them, your family, friends, and this program will be cheering you on. For all of the anxiety, uncertainty, and fatigue that you will encounter, the early years of your career are going to be among the most exciting of your life. Relish these years, no matter how challenging they may be.

Don't let technology remove the human element of healthcare in your desire for efficiency. The goal here is to give you more time for human contact and to listen. Every patient's story is important to hear.

There will also be times when you may not be particularly happy with the patients or the other people around you. During these times, the key will be for you to never lose sight of the fact that taking care of patients and their families is a privilege that you have earned through your dedication and efforts. At the end of the day, you will find that all of your reasons will lead you back to people and to that hole in your heart.

Become part of the debate. Take time to teach. Take time to explain. Speak out. But most importantly in the work you do every day, dare to believe in what is possible and instill in others this same sense of possibility. It will take daring, because optimism is a choice; detachment is an easier path. So do more than dare to explore or discover; dare also to lead.

One last request: please remember that you were once students, how that felt, and what you needed. We hope that you will become part of the solution, that you will continue to grow personally and professionally, and that you will mentor others in a culture of international caring. George Bernard Shaw once remarked that "life is a sort of splendid torch to hold up, to make burn as brightly as possible before handing it on to future generations." For you graduates, the torch is your nursing pin. It symbolizes the power in each and every one of you to create a quality of life, and to face change squarely and with integrity, confident that you are being true to principle and purpose.

Welcome to a healing profession. You are nurses. From here, wherever you may go, never forget that this is what you help to do. This is your greatest power, your greatest gift. Congratulations for your commitment, for challenges conquered, for projects completed, for goals reached and even surpassed. Tonight, enjoy your family and friends, and celebrate this very special moment in time. Go in joy and peace. Best wishes to you, graduates!

References

Algoso, M., Ramjan, L., East, L., & Peters, K. (2024). Teaching and learning the art of nursing through aged care work experience. *Teaching & Learning in Nursing*, *19*(1), e89–e95.

American Association of Colleges of Nursing. (2023). *Nursing workforce fact sheet.*

American Association of Colleges of Nursing. (2024). *Nursing faculty shortage fact sheet.*

Antig, A., Arañez, S., Cañazares, C., & Palompo, D. (2024). Nursing faculty shortage impact on nursing students: A descriptive phenomenological study. *Nursing Research and Practice*, *24*, 1–10, Article ID 1751942. https://doi.org/10.1155/2024/1751942

Barker, E. (2006). Mentoring: A complex relationship. *Journal of the American Academy of Nurse Practitioners, 18,* 56–61.

Benner, P. (2001). *From novice to expert: Excellence and power in clinical nursing practice.* Prentice Hall.

Brown, R., Da Rosa, P., Pravecek, B., & Carson, P. (2023). Factors associated with changes in nurses' emotional distress during the COVID-19 pandemic. *Applied Nursing Research: ANR*, *69*, 151659. https://doi.org/10.1016/j.apnr.2022.15165

Chichester, M. (2009). Passing the torch: Teaching the next generation of nurses. *Nursing for Women's Health, 13(6)*, 507–510.

Dempsey, L. (2007). The experiences of Irish nurse lecturers role transition from clinician to educator. *International Journal of Nursing Education Scholarship, 4*(1), 1–12.

Erikson, E. H. (1950). *Childhood and society*. W. W. Norton.

Haddad, L. M., Annamaraju, P., & Toney-Butler, T. J. (2023). *Nursing Shortage.* StatPearls Publishing. https://www.ncbi.nlm.nih.gov/books/NBK493175/

Haigh, C., & Johnson, M. (2007). Attitudes and values of nurse educators: An international survey. *International Journal of Nursing Education Scholarship, 4*(1), 1–11.

Health Resources and Services Administration. (2026, February). *Apply to the Nurse Corps loan repayment program.* https://bhw.hrsa.gov/funding/apply-loan-repayment/nurse-corps

Homer. (1961).*Odyssey* (R. Fitzgerald, Trans.). Vintage.

Horton, B. (2003). The importance of mentoring in recruiting and retaining junior faculty. *AANA Journal, 71*(3), 189–195.

Johnson, R. (2007) In memoriam: Continuing my journey through project LEAD. *Association of Black Nursing Faculty, 18*(3), 76–77.

Khalid, N., Zapparrata, N., & Phillips, B. C. (2024). Theoretical underpinnings of technology based interactive instruction. *Teaching & Learning in Nursing*, *19*(1), e145–e149. https://doi-org/10.1016/j.teln.2023.10.004

Lee, M. (2024). Improving new graduate nurse retention with a transition to emergency nursing practice program. *Journal of Emergency Nursing, 50*, (2), 178–186.

Lewallen, L., Crane, P., Letvak, S., Jones, E, & Hu, J. (2003). An innovative strategy to enhance new faculty success.*Nursing Education Perspectives,* 3, 1–5. Retrieved May 20, 2027, from http://goliath.ecnext.com/free-scripts/document

National Center for Health Workforce Analysis. (2024). *State of the U.S. health care workforce, 2024.* Bureau of Health Workforce. https://bhw.hrsa.gov/sites/default/files/bureau-health-workforce/state-of-the-health-workforce-report-2024.pdf

National Council of State Boards of Nursing. (2021). *Report of findings from the 2021 RN nursing knowledge survey.*

National League for Nursing. (2005). *The scope and practice for academic nurse educators.*

National League for Nursing. (2006a). Statement: Mentoring of nurse faculty. *Nursing Education Perspectives*, 27(2), 110–113.

National League for Nursing. (2006b). *Nurse educators 2006: A report of the faculty census survey of RN and Graduate programs.*

National League for Nursing. (2006c) *Position statement: Mentoring of nurse faculty.*

NSI Nursing Solutions Inc. (2022). *2022 NSI national health care retention & RN staffing report. https://www.nsinursingsolutions.com/Documents/Library/NSI_National_Health_Care_Retention_Report.pdf*

Rosseter, R. (2024, April). *Nursing workforce fact sheet. American Association of Colleges of Nursing.* https://www.aacnnursing.org/news-data/fact sheets/nursing./

Rush K., Janke, R., Duchscher, J., Phillips, R., & Kaur, S. (2019). Best practices of formal new graduate transition programs: An integrative review. *International Journal of Nursing Students, 94*, 139–158. https://doi.org/10.1016/j.ijnurstu.2019. 02.010

Sanders, D., & Welk, D. (2005). Strategies to scaffold learning: Applying Vygotsky's zone of proximal development. *Nurse Educator, 30*(5), 203–207.

Silas, B., & Kleiner, C. (2001). Novice faculty: Encountering expectations in academia. *Journal of Advanced Nursing, 43 (1),* 206–215.

Smiley, R., Ruttinger, A., Oliveira, C., Hudson C., Allgeyer, L., Reneau, R., Silvestre, K., & Alexander, M. (2020). The national nursing workforce survey. *Journal of Nursing Regulation*, *12*(1), S1–S96.

Smiley, R. A., Allgeyer, R. L., Shobo, Y., Lyons, K. C., Letourneau, R., Zhong, E., Kaminski-Ozturk, N., & Alexander, M. (2023). *The 2022 national nursing workforce survey. Journal of Nursing Regulation, 14*(1), S1–S90.

Tamata, A. T., & Mohammadnezhad, M. (2023). A systematic review study on the factors affecting shortage of nursing workforce in the hospitals. *Nursing Open*, *10*(3), 1247–1257. https://doi.org/10.1002/nop2.1434

Thorpe, K., & Kalischuk, R. (2003). A collegial mentoring model for nurse educators. *Nursing Forum, 38*(1), 5–15.

■ CHAPTER 10

Building a Culture of Safety

If you put good people in bad systems, you get bad results. You have to water the flowers you want to grow.

—Stephen Covey

Introduction

Civility refers to the actions of polite behavior toward others, ensuring that their dignity is maintained. Civil behavior demonstrates respect and courtesy toward others (Atashzadeh Shoorideh et al., 2021). In healthcare, civility is essential for creating a culture of trust and open communication among providers. A culture of civility ensures a positive work environment, improves job satisfaction, and enhances patient care.

Building a culture of safety in nursing is essential to ensure a collaborative and supportive environment. However, this endeavor comes with professional challenges and a significant amount of stress when nurses face current realities: staffing concerns, long work hours, and the increasing demands of complex patient care. Communication breakdown and conflicting expectations among health care providers can lead to misunderstandings and increased tension. Efforts to address and manage these pressures are daunting, and can create an environment ofincivility, which threatens health providers' primary goal of delivering safe, quality patient care (Angelo, 2019).

Anderson and Pearson (1999) define incivility as "negative behaviors with low-intensity and unclear intention that damage the targeted person." Associated terms include lateral violence, workplace violence, bullying, and aggression. Factors triggering incivility events can involve communication barriers (nurse to patient; nurse to nurse, nurse to physician), staffing issues (patient-to-nurse ratios), lack of resources (basic needs, technology, equipment), safety (bullying, workplace violence), and life events (personal or family concerns, lack of sleep, burnout, compassion fatigue). They are often interrelated and contribute to time constraints, missed care and increased stress for all involved (Algoso et al., 2023).

The Fallout From Incivility

Workplace Violence

Any harmful act, physical, sexual, or psychological, committed against nurses in the workplace by a patient or visitor is termed "workplace violence" (WPV; Kafle et al., 2022). Estimated to involve 95% of workers, WPV presents a considerable risk for both workers and employers (National Council of State Boards of Nursing, 2021; NSI Nursing Solutions Inc., 2025). Violence on the job can impact workers' lives in the measure of lost income, increased health care costs, and missed days of work. Also, violence affects nurse-patient ratios for those nurses managing heavier clinical care workloads.

Research by Atashzadeh Shoorideh et al. (2021) found that over 40% of all nurses experience some form of workplace violence.The authors report that the majority of emergency department nurses have been confronted with verbal abuse, while over 80% have been subjected to physical violence. Protests by both professionals and the public to stem violent acts against health care workers have not resulted in a reduction in these events. Authors Spelten et al. (2020) question whether violence against workers is becoming "the new normal."

Burnout and Compassion Fatigue

Personal stressors can heighten the strain on nurses' health, life-work balance, and overall job satisfaction, leading to difficulties in professional performance. Financial and family responsibilities and challenges can impact decision-making on the job. This struggle to achieve a work-life balance can lead to absenteeism, disengagement, or "presenteeism," where nurses are physically but not mentally present (Angelo, 2019). Physical and emotional exhaustion can result in complete role "burnout," a major factor driving nurses from their careers. These stressors often leave nurses feeling overworked, exhausted, and degraded.

As a form of burnout, "compassion fatigue" occurs in response to traumatic experiences. The trauma felt can be identified as primary (experiencing mental or physical harm), or secondary (witnessing an individual's suffering). Nurses are especially vulnerable to developing compassion fatigue from continual exposure to the suffering of others. They become overwhelmed with this constant distress. yet continue to work, dismissing their own personal suffering (Todaro-Franceschi, 2015).

Wolotira (2023) proposes that burnout is a consequence of compassion fatigue, yet the two are distinct experiences. Burnout tends to have a gradual onset, whereas compassion fatigue may present more rapidly or suddenly. Burnout is often characterized by feelings of hopelessness, emotional exhaustion, lack of self-efficacy, and decreased productivity in the workplace. Precipitated by long-standing exposure to workplace stressors, Wolotira's work reveals that burnout occurs in 40%–75% of health care professionals.

In areas where there is a higher incidence of death, suffering is more visible, putting larger numbers of nurses at risk. According to Todaro-Franceschi (2019), a common response *to* suffering *is* suffering. Those nurses employed in critical care, trauma, oncology, hospice, emergency, and intensive care units are at high risk for compassion fatigue. During the pandemic, nurses who cared for COVID patients experienced this trauma at overwhelmingly high levels.

Bullying

Negative outcomes of incivility lead to detachment, decreased work productivity, sleep pattern disorders, physical and mental health illnesses. Sensitized and overwhelmed, these individuals can become "victims" of bullying. The American Nurses Association (ANA) defines bullying as "repeated, unwanted harmful actions intended to humiliate, offend and cause distress in the recipient" (ANA, 2019). Bullying behaviors range from unrealistic workload assignments, exclusion by coworkers, and public criticism (Hampton & Rayens, 2019; Smith et al., 2020) to physical violence and death threats. It is important to understand that bullying is a serious problem that cannot be ignored, as it can rapidly escalate the stress experienced, and the impact on the bullied victim creates a vicious cycle of negative self-worth and self-confidence which ultimately compromises patient safety (Edmonson & Zelonka, 2019).

Unfortunately, bullied individuals endure the abuse by continuing to work in this toxic setting. Without support, they become silent, distrustful of others, and fear getting help. The cycle continues, compromising safety and raising the potential for "adverse events" such as missed care, patient falls, or medication errors. Heavy workloads, vulnerability to injuries from scarce staffing and a workplace environment of incivility contribute heavily to the "poor professional quality of life for nurses" (Todaro-Franceschi, 2019).

Over time, these factors affect one's personal health, lower job satisfaction, and contribute to a decline in workplace morale, teamwork, and the overall quality of care (Schlak et al., 2021). The cumulative toxic effects of personal, professional, and environmental stressors negatively impact individual performance. They combine to create a pattern of poor performance in other employees, affecting and "infecting" the entire unit (Angelo, 2019).

Workplace violence has been cited as a significant reason for nursing "turnovers," a designated term for those newlygraduated nurses hired to work, often in specialty units (ICU/ED) who leave their positions within the first two years. The lack of a formal, standard education/ orientation program, administered over a designated time period upon employment to a nursing position, has been linked to feelings of incompetence and lack of support. Moreover, increased turnover rates often necessitate hiring contract nurses, who typically work for a set period of time, and with a higher rate of base pay (Lee, 2024). With healthcare becoming more complex, and new nurses lacking confidence to practice, organizations are finding an increasing need for transition to practice (TTP) programs.

Upholding Civility Within the Profession of Nursing

Strategies for Success: Creating a Blame-Free Environment

Establishing and maintaining civility within healthcare is an essential component of preventing or reducing errors and improving overall health care quality. Creating and sustaining a "just" culture of safety is necessary in order to anticipate, identify, evaluate, and strategize solutions. Components of such a culture include establishing a blame-free environment, encouraging teamwork, promoting transparency, and increasing interprofessional collaboration (Hons et al., 2022). The ANA (2025) Code of Ethics for Nurses guides nurses in professional expectations regarding workplace behaviors among colleagues. The code assists nurses in handling challenging ethical issues to guarantee the delivery of safe and professional care

Interprofessional collaboration is vital to communicating the need for optimal patient-centered care in the pursuit of building and maintaining a civil culture. An effective team is one where all members (including patients) unite to share their observations, expertise, and decision-making responsibilities. To achieve civility, the team demonstrates integrity, trust, and respect toward its members (Gluyas, 2015).

Creating a blame-free environment is fundamental to a culture of safety and increases error reporting among staff. A blame-free atmosphere offers a safe and transparent space to voice any concerns, which ultimately improves patient outcomes. Staff blame or reprimanding will likely halt reporting errors, which poses the risk of more harm. The acknowledgment of error leads to the creation of a learning organization in which staff learns from patient safety events. This is essential for continuous quality improvement and decreased chance of error repetition.

Recognizing Stressors

Personal stressors can significantly impact nurses' health, life/work balance, and overall job satisfaction, leading to gaps in professional performance (Hampton & Rayens, 2019). The demands of physical and emotional exhaustion from managing personal and professional challenges may lead to burnout, affecting concentration and decision-making abilities. Other personal issues may arise if bullying is experienced in the workplace, which can lead to negative self-worth and self-confidence. This can compromise patient safety, as nurses may be more prone to have errors in medication administration or when making clinical decisions. Additionally, the struggle to maintain a healthy family/work balance can lead to absenteeism, disengagement, or presenteeism, where nurses are physically present but mentally not present (Angelo, 2019). Over time, these factors lower job satisfaction and may contribute to a decline in workplace morale, teamwork, and the overall quality of care. The cumulative effects of these personal stressors not only negatively impact individual performance but can also create a pattern of poor performance in other employees and affect the entire unit.

Person-Centered Care

According to Roger's "person-centered care" theory, positive and open relations between the nurse and patient are central to effective care. Roger believed individuals can achieve personal growth through unconditional positive regard within trusting, genuine, and open relationships (Duphily, 2022). In order to form a trusting relationship, the nurse must apply therapeutic communication and incorporate active listening. Trust increases the patient's amount of information shared to enable a more detailed and complete assessment. These actions ultimately empower patients to make informed decisions and become active participants in their care. Incorporating the values and beliefs of the culture of safety with patients increases the patient's experience, the accuracy of diagnoses, and the inclusive plan of care to permit safe and patient-centered care.

Promoting civility in healthcare is essential to cultivate a positive, respectful, and collaborative environment where both staff, family members and patient relations thrive (Angelo, 2019). Civility begins with open, honest communication, where family members and patients trust health care team members as they express concerns and ideas without fear of retaliation or judgment (Pavlish et al., 2020).

The Role of Nursing Leadership in Establishing and Maintaining Civility

In mediating any act of incivility within their health care organizations, nurse leaders are crucial in promoting and maintaining a respectful atmosphere among staff. With clear protocols in place, and an understanding of the culture within the organization, nursing leaders have the ability to create a safe, civil work environment where employees feel safe, have the ability to be heard, and freedom to deliver safe, informed quality care (Atashzadeh Shoorideh et al., 2021).

Civility builds the foundation for effective communication, collaboration, and mutual respect, which are all crucial for delivering high-quality patient care. By encouraging empathy, active listening, and professional accountability, nursing leaders help relieve stress, prevent burnout, and mitigate conflicts, creating a more cohesive and positive environment. When nurses feel respected and valued, job satisfaction increases, leading to improved performance, reduced turnover, and improved patient outcomes (Hons et al., 2022).

Building a culture of safety in health is essential for protecting patients and staff. Hospitals and clinics can be demanding environments where health care professionals are expected to make high-stakes decisions under extreme pressure. Mistakes can lead to severe consequences that affect not only patient outcomes but also the welfare of nurses and other health care workers.

Maintaining a culture of civility in nursing represents the shared values, beliefs, and attitudes that everyone in a health care setting holds toward safety. This culture emphasizes a commitment to minimizing harm for both patients and staff. It means that safety is not just an individual's responsibility but a collective effort across the entire health care team. A culture of safety is a set of shared perceptions and values that create a commitment to safety within a health care facility. In nursing, this culture is critical because nurses are on the front lines of patient care. They are often the first to notice changes in a patient's condition, identify safety concerns, and take action to prevent potential problems.

With a strong safety culture in place and leadership support, nurses feel empowered to speak up, knowing that their input is valued and that they will not face negative repercussions for reporting errors. This culture creates an environment where health care professionals work together, openly communicate, and continuously seek to improve safety practices. A culture of safety goes beyond protecting patients from immediate harm. It also influences the overall quality of health care delivery. Additionally, a safe environment contributes to the well-being and job satisfaction of health care staff, reducing burnout and turnover rates.

Learning From Adverse Events

Health care is constantly evolving, with new technologies, treatments, and procedures emerging. Continuous education and training help nurses and other health care professionals stay up to date on best practices and safety protocols. Educational programs that focus on error reporting, root cause analysis, and human factors are vital in building a culture of safety.

Nurses are accountable for the quality of their choices and actions. In the goal to deliver safe and accurate care, mistakes, or adverse events, may occur. In the event of an error, the nurse is required to report the occurrence and any consequences. Reporting mistakes in health care delivery is vital in order to implement appropriate interventions and repair the error. The information provided from adverse events can be used to address system flaws that contribute to patient safety events.

Creating a just culture means focusing on learning rather than blaming. In such a culture, errors are viewed as learning opportunities instead of occasions for punishment. This approach encourages staff to speak up about safety issues and helps build a climate of trust. Nurses, doctors, and other health care professionals are more likely to take ownership of their roles in maintaining safety when they know that their efforts will be supported rather than criticized.

Leaders should focus on creating a just culture where the goal is not to punish individuals for mistakes but to understand the underlying safety issues and prevent similar incidents in the future. By openly discussing errors and safety concerns, health care teams can develop strategies to improve patient safety and reduce medical errors over time.

A supportive work environment is vital for maintaining a strong culture of safety. When health care workers feel supported by their leaders and peers, they are more likely to engage in behaviors that promote patient safety. For example, leaders can establish programs that recognize and reward staff members who actively participate in safety initiatives. This recognition not only boosts morale but also reinforces the importance of a safe work environment.

Tools Fostering Safety and Civility

Nurses can anticipate and intervene in potentially high-risk patient situations by integrating structured communication models into daily practice with the use of "handoff reports." When reporting on their assigned patients to oncoming shift personnel, nurses report that these tools enable them to prioritize possible problems (Gluyas, 2015).

Bedside shift reporting (BSR) involves the nurse giving handoff in the same room with the patient. BSR can utilize situation, background, assessment, and recommendation (SBAR) or I-PASS to provide the patient with a consistent message while increasing interaction. This promotes trust, compliance, and active participation with the plan of care (Duphily, 2022). Integrating these tools can enhance communication to foster safer patient care.

SBAR is one example that offers a clear, timely, and efficient method to convey information to providers and other nurses. This communication tool maintains common language among team members, aids in shared decision-making and conflict resolution, and ultimately improves patient satisfaction and outcomes (Duphily, 2022).

The mnemonic I-PASS (illness severity, patient summary, action list, situation awareness/contingency plans, and synthesis) is an additional communication tool (Blazin et al., 2020). To evaluate the effectiveness of I-PASS, the authors carried out a quality improvement initiative by implementing I-PASS in handoff contexts. The study found that I-PASS utilization by health care professionals contributed to decreased error rates and improved handoff performance (Blazin et al., 2020), thus reducing potential conflict.

Technology can significantly enhance system safety performance. Electronic health records, for example, can help track patient information and reduce medication errors by providing accurate, up-to-date data. Safety event reporting systems can also document incidents and analyze trends, making it easier to identify areas needing improvement.

Using data to monitor safety trends enables health care organizations to make informed decisions about safety protocols and safety improvements. For example, data analytics can help health care teams understand potential risk factors and develop strategies to address them. Investing in technologies that support patient safety can make a significant difference in the overall health care quality.

Finding Balance: Combating Burnout and Compassion Fatigue

Remaining true to the genuine caring nature of the profession, keeping foremost in one's mind the meaning and purpose of the role, helps nurses to recognize, respond and recover from the clutches of compassion fatigue. One strategy for those in nursing leadership roles is to view compassion fatigue and burnout as "on-the-job injuries." As well, mental health resources such as employee assistance programs in the workplace should be enabled (Wolotira, 2023). The ART model (Todaro-Franceschi, 2015) is a self-awareness tool developed to help individual nurses and other caregivers enhance their quality of life. It includes the following:

- ***A***cknowledging a wound or feeling
- ***R***ecognizing choices and, with intention, choosing and taking purposeful action
- ***T***urning toward self and others to reconnect with ourselves and our environment in ways that foster contentment

Acknowledgment. Addressing one's own feelings, especially suffering, is a difficult but necessary step in order to enhance the professional quality of life and promote healing. As a reflective exercise, acknowledgment can guide nurses to become more aware of a situation and recognize whether there is a problem (how one acts/reacts with others, or an event that intensifies over the course of a shift). Exploring possible turning points can help establish those factors during work that may have contributed to an escalating incident. Reflection can help individuals pinpoint the moment when they began to feel this way.

Recognition. Depending on the situation, there may be many choices and actions that can be initiated. Some nurses may share their intended actions with a colleague. This helps to identify different perspectives or an alternative approach to resolve the conflict. If possible, giving the situation time is recommended before a final decision to proceed is made. Potential choices may include requesting critical incident stress debriefing, scheduling vacation time, or seeking employee assistance.

Turning. In this stage, individuals may step outside themselves to objectively examine their own self-care practices, including their general health status, eating, sleeping, and daily routines. In considering the presence of support systems; connections with patients, loved ones, and coworkers; and making time for the things most important in their lives, individuals are encouraged to express their feelings and articulate those aspects of their lives, away from work, that bring them joy and fulfillment.

The Durability of Resilience

Considered a valuable mechanism for survivors of trauma, resilience is the ability to recover from adversity. As a "trauma-informed" defense against daily stressors and challenges, resilience helps nurses to discover their coping skills, fostering therapeutic adaptation to the challenges of the professional role. In the process of developing resilience, nurses are encouraged to first address any personal adverse childhood events or stressors and their potential impact on patient care and treatment.

Many nurses have experienced trauma in their lives. A significant example can be found in their dedication to patients and families while working through the COVID-19 pandemic. In avoiding past trauma, coupled with current workplace stressors, nurses place themselves at high risk for experiencing compassion fatigue and burnout. Ultimately, the nurse is unable to carry out her work, and the quality of patient care suffers (Wolotira, 2023).

Leaders in the health care industry can positively affect the well-being of their nursing staff through a "trauma-informed" approach. Promotion of practices to decrease compassion fatigue and improve nurses' resilience, job satisfaction, and intent to stay in the position not only fosters individual self-care but provides a mentorship model in resilience for the benefit of future nurses. Wolotira (2023) states that further exploration of this topic is of such value that the Future of Nursing 2020–2030 Committee has included resilience in their work.

Reflective Questions

1. What has been your experience with incivility and conflict resolution?
2. How would you organize, strategize, and collaborate with others to address problems in the workplace?
3. What information would you need to collect? Skills needed? Obstacles faced?
4. What factors can encourage or discourage interdisciplinary teamwork?

Scenario

Incivility

With a track record of positive reviews and a recognized future leader by all who work with her, Rachel was promoted to the role of nurse manager of a 40-bed medical unit 3 months ago. She has worked on this unit since graduation from LPN school, returned for her ADN 5 years ago, and last year received her baccalaureate degree in nursing. Due to a recent reorganization, the hospital has experienced a change in nursing administration. Her current supervisor's approach contradicts both her democratic leadership style and the philosophy of her mentor, a supportive leader who has left the organization for a high level nursing management position in another city. Rachel has found the new supervisor to be authoritative and negative. When Rachel has attempted to discuss unit issues with her, her supervisor has replied that she was "too busy" and that Rachel "needed to develop a backbone." Yesterday, the supervisor told her that she must fire an outspoken nurse on the unit who had been openly expressing his frustration with the hospital's reorganization plan and the resultant disorganization on the unit. An industrious, well respected staff member, he has over 20 years of service to the organization.

Questions

1. As nurse manager, what is Rachel's next step?
2. If Rachel came to you, what would be your approach?
3. What questions would you ask? Factors to be considered?
4. Describe strategies for a resolution of this situation.

Food for Thought

The Sea Glass Story: A Metaphor for Durability of the Spirit

For whatever we lose (like a you or a me), it's always ourselves we find in the sea.

—E. E. Cummings

Sea glass, or "mermaid's tears," represents a symbol of transformation, resilience, and mystery. Each piece has undergone a journey, shaped and smoothed by the ocean's relentless waves. Challenges shape us. Each piece of sea glass represents healing and renewal, illustrating individual growth through its vibrant colors and polished edges. The uniqueness of sea glass highlights the importance of embracing imperfections (By the Sea Jewelry, n.d.).

The variety of sea glass colors are believed to have their own unique symbolism. Green sea glass is associated with healing, balance, and abundance, promoting both physical and emotional growth and renewal. Blue sea glass is linked to calmness, tranquility, and communication, enhancing self-expression and communication. White sea glass is related to purity, clarity, and new beginnings, which bring a sense of peace and calmness to mind and spirit. Believed to provide a sense of security and stability in times of change, brown sea glass is often connected to stability, grounding, and protection (Corcoran et al., 2010)

Sea glass serves as a reminder of our bond with nature, celebrating unity and interconnectedness through shared experiences. Each piece embodies hope and positivity, representing the wealth found in relationships and collective fulfillment rather than material possessions. Over years, waves and the sand change and shape the piece of glass into a smooth, beautiful colored gem, washed up onto the beach to be found. Many believe that sea glass carries positive energy and has the power to heal and bring peace. As a metaphor for change, the end product of glass thrown into the sea and tumbled about for ages, is a transformed treasure. Much like the journey sea glass takes, humans experiencing life's adversities shape us into the durable people we are and will become. For nurses, sea glass collecting teaches us valuable lessons—namely, to stop, look around and to appreciate nature to renew our senses of beauty, joy, peace, and awe. Also, through creative thinking initiated by a fresh vantage point (looking all around us), we acquire the tools to achieve new approaches (such as hobbies), the freedom of new perspectives, and ultimately satisfaction from ventures into the unknown. Sea glass symbolizes transformation, embodying resilience and the beauty that arises from overcoming life's challenges and hardships. Sea glass grew out of a rainy-day family past time of collecting and wire-wrapping Caribbean sea glass. From years of beach combing, we gathered pieces of sea glass, using our imagination to create different forms of art from these gems. Each design is made from items found mostly along the shores of Caribbean beaches, collected through travel. No two creations are ever alike since each piece of sea glass or pottery is different.

Appreciating Authentic Sea Glass

Value—Sea glass will only increase in value as supplies diminish.

Genuine—Sea glass cannot be replicated by artificial means.

Made by Nature—It cannot be mass produced.

Unique—Each piece is truly "one of a kind."

Provenance—It has a history, a story.

Sea Glass Is Natural—It is not altered, reshaped, artificially etched, or colorized.

Made by the Sea—It is naturally tumbled in the ocean for many years.

Eco-friendly—Once trash now treasure, sea glass and has no by-product.

Tactile—Real sea glass has an amazing texture that seems to soothe.

Handcrafted—Real sea glass jewelry is artisan made.

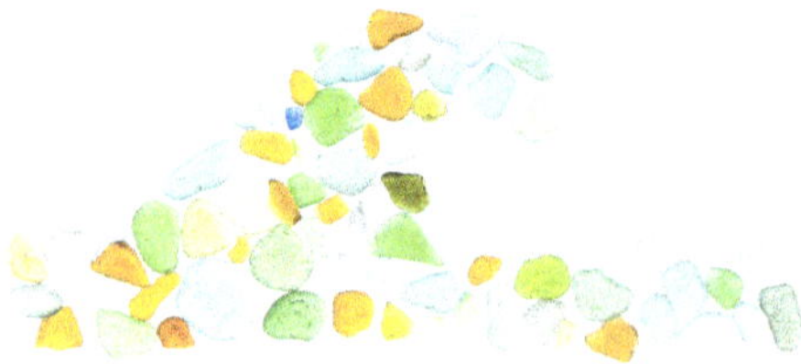

Image 10.1

The Sea Glass Poem by Bernadette Noll[1]

I want to age like sea glass.

Smoothed by the tides, but not broken.

Life's currents tumble me over years, softening my hard edges

I ride the waves, and the tide's impact tosses me on the shore, between rocks

I rest until I have the strength to do what is next.

The next wave carries me to the place I am supposed to land.

I connect with others, who bring me along on their own path

New possibilities are presented, new ideas are born.

People see what I have become, embracing all that I am

Appreciating my nature, they hold me gently

Awed by the patina, neither flashy nor dull,

but just the right finish.

References

American Nurses Association. (2019). *Position statement: Incivility, bullying, and workplace violence*. https://www.nursingworld.org/practice-policy/nursing-excellence/official-position-statements/id/incivility-bullying-and-workplace-violence/

American Nurses Association. (2025). *Code of ethics for nurses*. American Nurses Publishing. https://codeofethics.ana.org/home

Anderson, L. M., & Pearson, C. M. (1999). Tit for tat? The spiraling effect of incivility in the workplace. *The Academy of Management Review, 24*(3), 452–471.

Angelo, E. (2019). Managing interpersonal conflict: Steps for success. *Nursing Management, 50*(6), 22–28.

Atashzadeh Shoorideh, F., Moosavi, S., & Balouchi, A. (2021). Incivility toward nurses: A systematic review and meta-analysis. *Journal of Medical Ethics and History of Medicine*, *14*, 15.

1. Adapted selections from Bernadette Noll, "I Want To Age Like Sea Glass," https://www.huffpost.com/entry/i-want-to-age-like-sea-glass_b_5317199. Copyright © 2014 by Bernadette Noll.

Blazin, L. J., Sitthi-Amorn, J., Hoffman, J. M., & Burlison, J. D. (2020). Improving patient handoffs and transitions through adaptation and implementation of I-pass across multiple handoff settings. *Pediatric Quality & Safety, 5*(4). https://doi.org/10.1097/pq9.0000000000000323

By the Sea Jewelry. (n.d.). *What is sea glass of beach glass*. Retrieved March 22, 2025, from https://bytheseajewelry.com/what-is-sea-glass-or-beach-glass/

Corcoran, P. L., Packer, K., & Biesinger, M. C. (2010). First-cycle grain weathering processes: Compositions and textures of sea glass from Port Allen, Kauai. *Journal of Sedimentary Research, 80*(10), 884–894. https://doi.org/10.2110/jsr.2010.077

Duphily, N. (2022). *Moving from your associate to your baccalaureate nursing degree* (1st ed.). Cognella Academic Publishing.

Edmonson, C., & Zelonka, C. (2019). Our own worst enemies: The nurse bullying epidemic. *Nursing Administration Quarterly, 43*(3), 274–279. https://doi.org/10.1097/NAQ.0000000000000

Gluyas, H. (2015). Effective communication and teamwork promotes patient safety. *Nursing Standard, 29*(49), 50–57. https://doi.org/10.7748/ns.29.49.50.e10042

Hampton, D., & Rayens, M. K. (2019). Impact of psychological empowerment on workplace bullying and intent to leave. *JONA: Journal of Nursing Administration, 49*(4), 179–185.

Hampton, D., & Rayens, M. K. (2021). Impact of psychological empowerment on workplace bullying and intent to leave. *JONA: The Journal of Nursing Administration, 51*, S41–S47. https://doi-org.fitchburgstate.idm.oclc.org/10.1097/NNA.0000000000001075

Hons, M. O., Lam, L., & Gilbert, J., & Hills, D. (2022). Nurse leadership in promoting and supporting civility in health care settings: A scoping review. *Journal of Nursing Management, 30*(8), 4221–4233. https://doi.org/10.1111/jonm.13883

Kafle, S., Paudel, S., Thapaliya, A., & Acharya, R. (2022). Workplace violence against nurses: A narrative review. *Journal of Clinical and Translational Research, 8*(5), 421–424.

Lee, M. (2024). Improving new graduate nurse retention with a transition to emergency nursing practice program. *Journal of Emergency Nursing, 50*(2), 178–186.

National Council of State Boards of Nursing. (2021). NCSBN's environmental scan COVID-19 and its impact on nursing and regulation. *Journal of Nursing Regulation,11*(4), S1–S36. https://doi.org/10.1016/s2155-8256(21)00002-8

NSI Nursing Solutions Inc. (2025). *2025 NSI national health care retention and RN staffing report.* https://www.nsinursingsolutions.com/Documents/Library/NSI_National_Health_Care_Retention_Report.pdf

Pavlish, C. L., Henriksen, J., Brown-Saltzman, K., Robinson, E. M., Warda, U. S., Farra, C., Chen, B., & Jakel, P. (2020). A team-based early action protocol to address ethical concerns in the intensive care unit. *American Journal of Critical Care: An Official Publication, 29*(1), 49–61.

Schlak, A. E., Aiken, L. H., Chittams, J., Poghosyan, L., & McHugh, M. (2021). Leveraging the work environment to minimize the negative impact of nurse burnout on patient outcomes.*International Journal of Environmental Research and Public Health, 18(*2), 610. https://doi.org/10.3390/ijerph18020610

Smith, C. R., Palazzo, S. J., Grubb, P. L., & Gillespie, G. L. (2020). Standing up against workplace bullying behavior: Recommendations from newly licensed nurses. *Journal of Nursing Education and Practice, 10*(7), 35. https://doi.org/10.5430/jnep.v10n7p35

Spelten, E., Thomas, B., O'Meara, P., van Vuuren, J., & McGillion, A. (2020). Violence against emergency department nurses: Can we identify the perpetrators? *PLoS ONE, 15*(4), e0230793. https://doi.org/10.1371/journal.pone.0230793

Todaro-Franceschi, V. (2015). The ART of maintaining the "care" in healthcare. *Nursing Management, 46*(6), 53–55. https://doi.org/10.1097/01.NUMA.0000465407.76450.ab

Todaro-Franceschi, V. (2019). *Compassion fatigue and burnout in nursing: Enhancing professional quality of life* (2nd ed.). Springer Publishing.

Wolotira, E. A. (2023). Trauma, compassion fatigue, and burnout in nurses: The nurse response. *Nurse Leader, 21*(2), 202–206. https://doi.org/10.1016/j.mnl.2022.04.009

Figure Credit

IMG 10.1: Copyright © 2017 Depositphotos/Tamara_k.

CHAPTER 11

Cultural Literacy

People of different religions and cultures live side by side in almost every part of the world, and most of us have overlapping identities which unite us with very different groups. We can love what we are, without hating what—and who—we are not. We can thrive in our own tradition, even as we learn from others, and come to respect their teachings.

—Kofi Annan, Former Secretary-General of the United Nations

Introduction

Nurses encounter a wide variety of patients throughout the course of their career. Considering the United States' diversity in race and ethnicity (World Health Organization, 2022), it can be assumed that providers' knowledge of cultural differences is vital to ensuring that all individuals are afforded health care services that align with their specific needs. Cultural differences are those traditions, beliefs and values held within a particular culture. Cultural, ethnolinguistic, and racial diversity has profound implications for nursing practice. Incorporating cultural awareness into the plan of care enables a nurse to respond appropriately to the specific needs of diverse patients and avoids incidents where patients from minority groups experience lower-quality care (Červený et al., 2022). Awareness of cultural differences affecting patient care creates the ability to understand the perspectives of others in delivering informed, current, and holistic patient-centered care (Kaihlanen et al., 2019).

Cultural Dissonance

Cultural dissonance is an experience of unfamiliarity with the people, places, or things due to customs, values, beliefs, or language. It is a sense of conflict when one confronts different cultural values, beliefs, or practices, primarily noted in relation to race, ethnicity, age, religion, class, physical ability, or sexual orientation. This phenomenon often arises in multicultural environments, impacting communication and social interactions, making awareness of cultural differences crucial for harmony (Suárez-Orozco & Suárez-Orozco, 2001).

Cultural dissonance in nursing occurs when nurses' cultural beliefs and practices clash with those of their patients, leading to communication barriers and misunderstandings that can potentially impact patient care. This occurrence can manifest in various ways, including differences in communication styles, interpretations of illness, and treatment preferences. For example, certain cultures use direct eye contact and open communication; other cultures may view this as a sign of disrespect. Similarly, many cultures have their own views regarding reasons and treatments for sickness, leading to differing opinions between patient and provider in the plan of care.

Religious beliefs, cultural traditions, and personal values can also influence a patient's preferences for treatment options that conflict with the providers' recommendations. Additionally, nurses must consider the needs of patients who rely on family practices traditions. Their decisions on health care interventions often clash with the provider's recommended plan of care.

Grewal et al. (2021) report that patients from different cultures experience disparities in care due to their providers' lack of knowledge of cultural diversity. Exacerbating this problem is a lack of diversity in health care leadership, the absence of culturally inclusive health care policies and procedures, and unfamiliarity with cultural literacy. From this misinterpretation, misunderstanding and miscommunication, the nurse-patient relationship suffers. When patients feel their cultural values are not respected, they become disenchanted with the system and noncompliant with treatment. Deteriorating miscommunication delays diagnosis and opportunities for intervention, causes emotional distress, and leads to unmet health outcomes and significant threats to patients' safety.

A lack of cultural understanding increases negative attitudes toward cross-cultural care and also affects health care professionals' perceived preparedness to take care of culturally diverse patients. Anxiety about interacting with people from different cultures influences a person's level of engagement in intercultural communication When combined with uncertainty, it further decreases effective communication and can lead to the increased use of stereotypes (Červený et al., 2022; Grewal et al., 2021).

Cultural Literacy

The importance of cultural literacy cannot be understated. It enables a nurse to deliver the highest quality, safest, and most patient-centered care possible. An accurate and thorough cultural assessment allows for the gathering of patient-specific cultural information. The pursuit of "culturally literate" care requires recognizing the various factors that can affect diversity and inclusion in nursing (McFarland & Wehbe-Alamah, 2019).

The foundation of providing culturally sensitive care rests on the transcultural nursing concept developed by nursing theorist Madeleine Leininger (McFarland & Wehbe-Alamah, 2019). Her work incorporates the cultural beliefs and practices of patients to support, maintain and regain health, or face end of life in a meaningful way.

Leininger's Theory of Culture Care: Diversity and Universality (1991)

Leininger states that healthcare cannot be effectively provided without considering the patient's cultural background. According to Leininger, culture is a fundamental component of human life and influences an individual's perception of health, illness, and healthcare (McFarland & Wehbe-Alamah, 2019). Therefore, health care providers must approach each patient with cultural sensitivity and strive to deliver care that is respectful and tailored to the patient's cultural needs. With cultural competency training as their framework, nurses support research for evidenced-based nursing practice. Educational nursing programs can develop curricula to prepare culturally competent nurses, while hospital organizations can employ the same framework to foster leadership and advanced practice.

By integrating a patient's cultural beliefs into the plan of care, nurses set the stage for the delivery of informed, holistic, individualized care. In their initial meeting, nurses introduce themselves to patients formally by using their title and last name. Following this introduction, the nurse asks the patient how they wish to be addressed, making it a point to record this information in the patient's chart. Nurses make sure to acknowledge any family members and visitors at the patient's bedside. Finally, recognizing and respecting social distancing, culturally sensitive nurses stand or sit at least an arm's length from the patient. They observe both patient and family members in regard to eye contact, touch, and nonverbal communication behaviors (Douglas et al., 2011).

If English is not the patient's primary language, a medical interpreter is typically contacted (with the patient's permission) before proceeding with interview questions, employing culturally sensitive and appropriate language (i.e. use of terms such as "unhoused" instead of "homeless"). Adopting a nonjudgmental approach shows respect for the patient's cultural beliefs, values, and practices. Whenever possible, integrating patients' cultural practices into their care supports and assures them that their cultural considerations are a priority

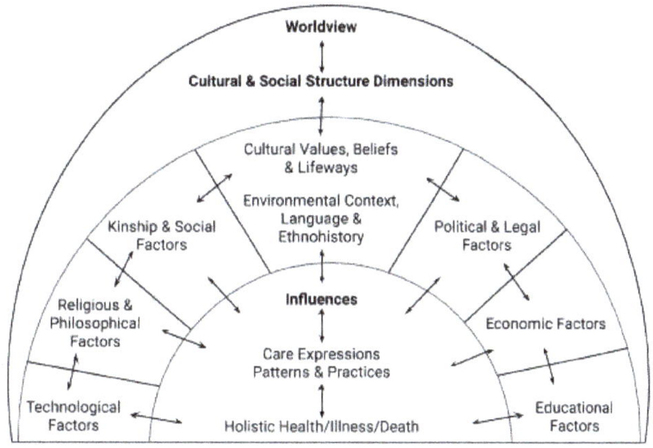

Figure 11.1 Leininger's Theory of Culture Care: Diversity and Universality
Created by Brian Duphily

Cultural Assessment: The "Four C's of Culture" Model

Initial steps in the introduction to the nurse-patient relationship include establishment of culturally sensitive environment. This can be achieved through incorporation of a cultural assessment when caring for all patients. One such tool is the "The Four C's of Culture Model," which poses questions about what the patient perceives, or *considers* to be, a problem; the *cause* of the problem; how they are *coping* with the problem; and how *concerned* they are about the problem (Galanti, 2014). This model employs the following questions:

- *What do you think is wrong? What is worrying you?* (What the patient *considers* to be the problem and how they refer to this problem.)
- *What do you think caused this problem? How did this happen?* (The patient believes this illness is a punishment *caused* by an offense.)
- *What are you doing to cope with this problem? How are you taking care of yourself?* (The patient *copes* by eating certain foods to treat the illness.)
- *How concerned are you? How serious is this problem for you? (The patient views the illness as being "God's will" and states, "It's in God's hands.")*

The freedom to express one's cultural beliefs is a fundamental right of all people. Nurses realize that people speak, behave, and act in many different ways due to the influential role that culture plays in their lives and their view of the world. Cultural literacy is a lifelong process of applying evidence-based nursing in agreement with the cultural values, beliefs, worldviews, and practices of patients to produce improved patient outcomes.

Culturally sensitive care requires nurses to combine their knowledge and skills with awareness, curiosity, and sensitivity about their patients' cultural beliefs. It takes motivation, time, and practice to develop cultural competence over one's nursing career. Culturally competent nurses have the power to improve the quality of care leading to better health outcomes for culturally diverse patients. Nurses who accept and uphold the cultural values and beliefs of their patients are more likely to develop supportive and trusting relationships with their patients. In turn, this opens the way for optimal disease and injury prevention and leads to positive health outcomes for all patients.

Cultivating Cultural Self-Awareness

Understanding oneself is a crucial step in forming a broader understanding and acceptance of other cultures (Lu & Wan, 2018). To develop such awareness, people can educate themselves about diverse cultures, learn to recognize and avoid stereotypes, and engage in cross-cultural communication and interaction. It is important to note that cultural awareness is an ongoing process that requires continuous learning and adaptation. Cultural self-awareness can help us understand what shapes our own values and beliefs and recognize our place in a larger multicultural society.

Acquiring cultural knowledge is another important step toward becoming a culturally competent nurse. The term cultural knowledge refers to seeking information about cultural health beliefs, history, customs, and values to understand patients' worldviews. To acquire cultural knowledge, the nurse actively seeks information about other cultures, including common practices, beliefs, values, and customs, particularly for those cultures that are established within the communities they serve. Cultural knowledge also includes understanding the historical backgrounds of culturally diverse groups in society, as well as physiological variations and the incidence of certain health conditions in culturally diverse groups. Cultural knowledge is best obtained through cultural encounters with patients from diverse backgrounds to learn about individual variations that occur within cultural groups (subcultures) and to prevent stereotyping.

Achieving cultural awareness takes time and effort. It requires frequent collaboration among providers, interpreters, patients, and families. Being part of the care "team" inspires patients to play a role in their own treatment plan. As active participants in care, patients have a voice. They are mutually respected members who feel seen, heard, and represented, empowered to advocate for themselves. An inclusive practice plan helps promote comprehensive health care practices to ensure that all patients, regardless of age, gender, race, sexual orientation, religion or background, receive the care they need. Collaboration improves the level of faith, trust and confidence among patients and providers. With strengthened patient-provider relationships, both groups can meet their expected outcomes.

Nurses can foster inclusivity in the following ways:

- **Cultural Awareness Education:** It is essential for health care institutions to include cultural awareness in their training programs; many states are requiring cultural competency education programs to prepare nurses and other health providers to communicate with patients from all backgrounds. This effort requires an ongoing process of continuous opportunities to reinforce and apply learning (Cai et al., 2021).
- **Cultural Assessments:** Upon admission, patient and nurse complete a "Cultural Assessment" tool to identify beliefs or values that may affect their care. This tool creates timely awareness of goals and expectations in developing the treatment plan. It fosters open dialogue and active listening. Completing the tool together fosters the need to include of language common to all, which equips provider, patient, and caregiver the ability to openly discuss issues and concerns. This assessment tool has the potential to further inclusivity "best practices" (Narayan & Mallinson, 2022).

- **Employment in Diverse Settings With Diverse Cultures:** Seeking such employment opportunities immerses nurses in the care of differing cultures, backgrounds, and religious beliefs. By actively working with patients who are different from themselves, nurses can self-reflect and raise their own awareness of potential biases and assumptions while improving their understanding of others' perspectives.
- **Advocacy for Inclusive Healthcare:** Communicating the importance of inclusive healthcare throughout the organization, from hiring practices to patient education materials, helps nurses align with these values and promotes a culture of inclusivity and respect. Nurses can become powerful advocates for their patients by lobbying for culturally sensitive policies and practices within health care facilities. These policies help protect patient needs and ensure nurses are able to safely and effectively provide all patients with personalized care (Williams et al., 2025).

There is a clear need to address the cultural literacy of health care professionals. It is essential to provide current, informed, and thoughtful training to health care professionals to raise their awareness of cultural differences and sensitize providers as to how culturally diverse patients are treated. Education builds awareness of cultural differences and helps to bridge the communication gap between language and culture among patients and health care providers. Cultural awareness guides nurses to prioritize inclusion efforts in planning care in order to better understand the impact a patient's cultural beliefs, heritage and traditions may have on their preferences. Equipped with a general perception and beliefs about an individual culture, a nurses' cultural world views can also raise their awareness regarding potential biases they may possess, ultimately improving overall patient outcomes and compliance with care.

Social Determinants of Health

The most beautiful people we have known are those who have known defeat, known suffering, known struggle, known loss, and have found their way out of those depths.

—Elisabeth Kübler-Ross

Social determinants of health (SDOH) involve those conditions into which people are born, grow, live, work, and age, along with the forces that affect and shape daily life (Olshansky, 2017). In their interactions with the health care industry, disadvantaged groups often face barriers, which are linked with those SDOH that limit their access to quality care and generate substantial health disparities (Valdez et al., 2023). These factors include socioeconomic status, environment (including air and water quality), food insecurity and food safety, education, employment, social networks, homelessness, and racism (Olshansky, 2017).

Low-income individuals, racial and ethnic minorities, rural residents, and the elderly often experience obstacles such as financial constraints, geographic isolation, cultural and language differences, and educational limitations. Other factors such as unstable housing, food insecurities, and systemic discrimination exacerbate these challenges, making it more difficult for them to navigate the health care system (Valdez et al., 2023).

It is often in the emergency department that this population meets their "first responder" lifeline in the form of the multitasking triage nurse, who has many expectations to fulfill in a short period of time. Equipped, experienced, and efficient, the resourceful triage nurse poses targeted assessment questions, prioritizes patient needs, and puts interventions in place to foster the patient's trust and compliance with the care they require.

The triage nurse identifies those individual barriers in the patient's assessment phase, which primarily addresses financial burdens, disabilities, psychological issues, and malnourishment. There may be language and educational obstacles, which contribute to a knowledge gap. A lack of transportation compounds the experience, decreasing access to healthcare, as well as exacerbating chronic and unmanaged medical conditions. Recognizing these inequities, it is the nurse who advocates and intervenes to connect patients with appropriate services and resources.

By understanding these barriers and the broader social and environmental factors influencing health outcomes, nurses can address health inequities and improve access to care for at-risk populations. There is strength in numbers, generating new ideas. Nurses can best help through developing partnerships. Collaborating with health care providers, policymakers, and community leaders can stimulate creative, innovative partnerships to promote health care access and improved outcomes.

To inform and prepare future nurses to address disparities in healthcare, SDOH content should be introduced and woven throughout entry level nursing curriculum through service-learning opportunities, classroom content, and clinical courses. This provides a valuable opportunity for nursing students to recognize the need to routinely assess and integrate SDOH into the plan of care. Ultimately, this exposure leads to graduate nurses who incorporate the role of change agent into their daily professional nursing practice (Olshansky, 2017).

Food Insecurity

Food insecurity is a critical SDOH that profoundly impacts individuals and communities. Affecting over 40 million Americans, this SDOH influences overall health outcomes, quality of life, and health care costs (Riley et al., 2020). Defined as the lack of consistent access to enough food for an active, healthy life, food insecurity can result from poverty, unemployment, lack of transportation, and inadequate access to grocery stores, particularly in underserved areas known as "food deserts" (Riley et al., 2020).

Limited access to nutritious food often leads to reliance on cheaper, calorie-dense, and nutrient-poor options, which can exacerbate health problems. Families that may have financial struggles turn to fast, processed foods, which are often more affordable, but lack essential vitamins and minerals. This dietary imbalance can contribute to obesity and related chronic conditions, creating a cycle of poor health that is difficult to break (Pronk et al., 2021).

Access to quality, affordable, and nutritious food is critical to promoting health across populations. However, food access remains a significant barrier to healthy eating in the United States today. Food deserts significantly impact the health of children and families. Low-income, communities of color, and urban communities are more at risk for experiencing food insecurity and poor diets. They are at a higher risk for obesity, diabetes, cardiovascular diseases, and mental health disorders. In those instances, nurses are critical in addressing important psychosocial questions to be able to intervene appropriately and provide adequate social services to these families.

The Supplemental Nutrition Assistance Program (SNAP) is one such plan which provides additional assistance during and after economic downturns (Mande & Flaherty, 2023). Approximately 62% of SNAP participants are families with children. SNAP offers nutritional support for working families with low-paying jobs, low-income older adults (60 years and older) and people with disabilities living on fixed incomes, as well as those households with low incomes. Nurses can help address food insecurity and access through identifying community risk and working to implement interventions such as farmer's markets that accept SNAP.

In conducting a nursing assessment for food insecurity, communication is key to establishing patient trust, choosing the correct screening method, and steering patients toward available resources (Riley et al., 2020). In their clinical education across many diverse settings, nursing students work with vulnerable populations across the life span. More than studying these concepts in a classroom or reading about them in a textbook, actual exposure to SDOH in the clinical setting teaches valuable lessons in communication, service, civic pride, cultural sensitivity, and critical thinking. Moreover, the experience leaves an indelible impression on those entering the nursing profession. Being informed on how to address these specific issues raises social awareness, offers a multitude of lifelong skills, and encourages interprofessional collaboration with health care providers, city and state officials, social work, public health, city planning, fire protection, and law enforcement public servants.

Healthy People 2030

Founded in 1980, the Healthy People organization created a framework to address and prioritize major health issues in the United States. The purpose of Healthy People is to identify and reduce health disparities by focusing on specific factors that affect an individual's health status. Initiatives include measurable public health objectives with ten-year targets to promote health and prevent disease within communities (Pronk et al., 2021).

Healthy People 2030 is a tool for health care providers to improve both the quality of the care they provide and the health of their patients and community. It provides a framework with evidence-based practice guidelines for a wide variety of common health care concerns, from hypertension to affordability. With 89% of the nurse practitioner (NP) population prepared in primary care and more than 75% actively practicing in primary care, NPs are uniquely positioned to help promote and achieve the Healthy People 2030 objectives (Office of Disease Prevention and Health Promotion, n.d.).

Past initiatives have been largely focused on individual health behaviors, and while the basic objectives for diabetes, heart disease, and obesity have been preserved from Healthy People 2020, the objectives of Healthy People 2030 have a new emphasis on health equity, SDOH, health literacy, and overall well-being, to ensure all populations can live healthier lives (Mager & Moore, 2020).

One of the most critical roles that nurses have in health promotion and disease prevention is that of an educator. Nurses spend a considerable amount of time with patients and are well-aligned to develop strong, trusting, long-term relationships. Connecting with patients to understand their individual risks and needs and providing them with personalized tools and resources to reduce their risks can greatly improve overall health and well-being (Mager & Moore, 2020).

Addressing SDOH is of particular importance for the well-being of communities, requiring nurses and nurse practitioners to provide resources and advocacy for economic stability, access to quality education, safe neighborhoods and built environments, and social context, They are well-positioned in the community to provide a wide range of services to at-risk populations, addressing the need for access to affordable healthcare and the prevention and management of chronic diseases, which is the foundation of Healthy People 2030.

Nursing can lead in translating SDOH awareness into action by incorporating Healthy People initiatives (Healthy People, 2030). SDOH are associated with negative health outcomes due to reduced resources and access to care. To achieve health equity, Healthy People initiatives should be integrated into current practice. Initiatives delineate measurable public health objectives with 10-year targets to promote health and prevent disease within communities (Pronk et al., 2021).

Holism

Holistic nursing care is an approach to patient care that considers social, spiritual, and psychological needs of patients (Albaqawi et al., 2021). Providing this all-inclusive care has been found to be an effective way to prevent diseases and death, as well as improve the quality of healthcare provided to patients (Algoso et al., 2024) However, despite its perceived benefits, research shows that the holistic approach is often overlooked. Moreover, many providers cite their lack of experience with holistic care, concentrating instead on patients' physical signs and symptoms, while disregarding spiritual, mental, and social needs (Ambushe et al., 2023)

In their research, authors Ambushe et al. (2023) found that many hospitals do not carry out the practice of treating the "whole" patient. According to surveys, 67% of patients in the United States do not receive holistic care. Data from other countries (Albaqawi et al., 2021) reveals health providers' overall lack of awareness with holistic care. The reports cited above give testament to the fact that holism, while key in treating the whole person, is often ignored. Ultimately, the neglect of this model and subsequent dismissal of holism in patient care is occurring internationally. By virtue of the fact that nurses in all settings of the discipline work closest to the patient on a daily basis, it seems remarkable that holistic care would be overlooked. By definition, holistic patient care is a comprehensive and compassionate approach to healthcare that prioritizes the whole individual rather than just treating isolated symptoms or conditions (Algoso et al., 2024).

In the education of nursing students, the long-term care clinical setting serves as a "holistic care training ground." This environment provides experiences that highlight the importance of human relationships and connectedness (Algoso et al., 20243). By understanding the interconnectedness of physical, emotional, social, spiritual, and environmental factors, nurses and other health care members can deliver holistic care that promotes overall health. The focus in this setting on patient-centered care, addressing SDOH, and cultivating a supportive and culturally sensitive environment are essential components of holistic nursing care.

Admittedly, there are realistic challenges to delivering holistic care in care settings: staffing shortages, high patient-to-nurse ratios, and limited resources. These factors contribute to time constraints and increased stress for care providers. These challenges may also inhibit the ability to provide individualized attention to residents of long-term care facilities, affecting the quality of care (Algoso et al., 2024). Moreover, the geriatric population's comorbidities and psychosocial needs can make it difficult to navigate the facets of patient management in this environment. Overall, the authors of the studies examined (Albaqawi et al., 2021; Algoso et al., 2024; Ambushe et al., 2023) came to similar conclusions. Lower levels of education, unit of work, lack of in-service- learning, quality of nurse-patient relationship, and a knowledge deficit regarding holistic care, were all associated with the current practice of holistic nursing care.

Recommendations for resolution of this problem would prioritize education. Collaboration among educational institutions and health care facilities for every individual affiliated with these health care organizations should be created using current evidence, with prioritized goals and continuously evaluated for their effectiveness. Formal in-service educational sessions could be conducted during employee orientation, with annual updates provided during required in-service education sessions or employee skills fairs. Partnerships with key players (nursing and other health care providers, local universities, and nursing education programs to research) could be developed to examine current evidence, discuss the problem. and strategize ways to create and implement holism into practice. The creation of a like-minded group made up of clinicians, educators, administration, students, and individuals from the community, vested in incorporating holistic care, is another important strategy to improve the knowledge and practice of holistic nursing care.

Reflective Questions

1. How has your culture shaped your life?
2. What information should your health provider know about your culture?
3. What are some things you've learned from interacting with people from other cultures?
4. Are you aware of any biases and assumptions about people with different values than you? If so, how do you handle these assumptions?
5. How do patients' SDOH (housing, food, culture, employment, socioeconomic status) affect their intent to seek healthcare?

Scenario

Addressing Cultural Responses to Pain

Following same-day cataract surgery, a 65-year old Asian patient has been refusing pain medication. He reports to the PACU (Post Anesthesia Care Unit) recovery room nurse that his pain is "bearable." When asked by the nurse to rate his pain level on a 0–10 scale, he is unable to supply a number. Thirty minutes later, the PACU nurse finds him restless, agitated, and uncomfortable. The nurse offers pain medication, and the patient continues to refuse, stating "I don't want to disturb you with my pain ... you have other patients who need you more."

Questions to Consider

1. What factors are involved in this patient's refusal of pain medication?
2. What should the nurse be aware of in regard to Asian cultural practices with care and treatment?
3. Do you think that this patient understands what is meant by a "pain scale," and how the 0–10 scale functions in assessing an individual's pain?
4. In this patient's mind, the needs of the nurse's other patients are more important. What other issues may affect this patient's care and treatment?
5. If a patient continues to refuse medication, should their wishes be respected?
6. How should the nurse proceed to meet this patients pain needs and his discharge outcomes?

Food for Thought

The Baby Boomer Culture: A Family Snapshot

Born between 1946 and 1964, the baby boomer generation has profoundly influenced culture, values, and economics. Representing more than a generational period in time, "boomers" personify 20th-century America, inspired by postwar success in the pursuit of personal freedom and purpose. They championed civil rights, gender equality, and environmental awareness, striving to create a fairer and more equitable society. This cultural shift influenced entertainment, fashion, language, and lifestyle, leaving a lasting legacy on global culture. Boomers continue reshaping society as they live longer, affecting changing concepts of family, work, aging, and community infrastructure along the way.

A Brief Snapshot: One Baby Boomer's "Cultural" Experience

Life during this time period can be accurately summarized by the word "change." We experienced change happening right before our eyes, particularly in the areas of technology, media, economics, and culture. We witnessed transformative social changes that still shape our world today. The following description hopefully provides the reader with some insight into these changes.

Before computers, we used our Olivetti Underwood/Smith Corona typewriters to submit school papers. Our hardworking librarian helped us to navigate the countless oak cabinets housing the "Dewey decimal" organizational system to research information for those papers we were composing.

Early on, we learned and practiced the "Palmer" method of penmanship. We were actually graded on how well we formed our letters. As a staid left-handed writer, I was "encouraged" to learn to the correct, "right-handed," acceptable way. It never took. At home, we were expected to use this training in handwriting skills to send thank-you cards (within 1 week) for ALL occasions.

Before cell phones, telephone "party lines" with neighbors was common practice. Imagine a family of four teenagers sharing one telephone line with the 90-year-old woman from across the street. Frequently we could hear our neighbor's breathing while she eavesdropped on my sisters' phone conversations with their boyfriends. "Someone" blew a whistle into the phone, and it solved the problem *toute de suite*.

Saturday mornings were spent gathered around the one TV set in the house (with four channels) watching cartoons, until our parents shooed us out for the day. *Popeye*, *Tom and Jerry*, *Bugs Bunny and Road Runner* were popular. Shows like *Lassie* (remember "Timmy fell down the well!"), *Sky King,* and *Flicka* were favorites. A rare event was being allowed to watch the nightmare-producing *Twilight-Zone* and *Alfred Hitchcock* shows.

With one television (black-and-white, no "clickers") and a "rabbit ears" antenna to get any of those four available TV channels, everyone in the family had to watch what my father, the designated "Channel Master," selected. The consummate prankster, he secretly pulled the plug while we were watching the Beatles debut on the *Ed Sullivan Show*, causing major pandemonium in the living room. He knew he had crossed the line with his four daughters. Seconds later, the television was back on; my dad proclaimed himself a hero by "fixing the TV." We never let him forget how close he was to a major injury that night. Meanwhile, I still have vivid memories of my grandfather, who shunned television, choosing instead to sit by the radio, listening to the Red Sox.

As we got older, we lived for Saturday afternoons with *Dick Clark's American Bandstand* and Sunday nights with Ed Sullivan. You could always be assured your favorite singer and/ or band would be featured on these shows at some point. With *American Bandstand*, we would stare at the teenagers dancing on the stage in their go-go boots, big hair, and miniskirts. We learned the dances of the era through them (the Twist, Swim, Locomotion, Frug, Mashed Potato) and tried them out at the Saturday night school dances and Battle of the Bands. We spent our allowance on "45s." These small records we kept safely stored in our own personal record player cases, so we could listen on end to our favorite singers in the privacy of our bedroom. Our transistor radios were always attached to us. We knew the DJ's (disc jockeys) names by heart. On a typical Saturday night, it was not unusual to call into the local radio station to request a song.

The power of television to reach the masses grew before our eyes in the '60s. We witnessed news firsthand. We remember hiding under our desks in our school basement during threats of nuclear war. We can readily recall where we were during the Cuban Missile Crisis, the assassinations of John F. Kennedy, Martin Luther King, and Robert Kennedy. We watched every event in the space program, especially the momentous walk on the moon. We lived with the Vietnam war, the protests, the riots, and the aftermath, displayed openly on the TV screen. As our parents and grandparents did and never really talked about, we experienced what it was like to lose loved ones to war.

Health practices were generally carried out in our home, using remedies from our English ancestors. My grandmother sprinkled salt in our shoes or boots on cold days to keep our feet warm when walking to school. She was also a proponent of castor oil for whatever ailed anyone. Vicks VapoRub was also used with great abandon for every malady under the sun. For our parents and grandparents, it seemed to be their first line of defense. They must have had stock in the Vicks corporation. My mother or grandmother would typically apply a liberal amount of the pungent ointment on our chests, followed by a piece of flannel beneath our shirts. Everyone at school knew you had been sick, as the smell never left you for days.

Trips to the hospital were a last resort. My mother had taken a first aid course in 1941, and the well-worn manual was a popular reference. Along with the phrase to "tough it out," mercurochrome, hydrogen peroxide, and Band-Aids replaced stitches on scrapes and cuts.

For transportation, we lived in the city and walked (safely) everywhere or took the city bus for trips "downtown" on special occasions or medical appointments. We had one car in a family of five kids, two parents, and two grandparents. Cars were big enough back then to house a small family. Seat belts were rare. I have memories of "steering the car" while sitting on my dad's lap as he drove or being squashed between my siblings and cousins as we bounced over the beach road seated on the tailgate of a moving station wagon. Meanwhile, my newborn baby brother slept soundly in his unrestrained "car bed" in the back seat. Favorite trips were to the beach every weekend, at the bargain price of $5 a carload. "Drive-in" theaters cost $6 a carload, and yes, we actually stuffed friends in the trunk to save money.

Recycling took on a different meaning for this boomer family. All of our toys and clothes, in good condition and no longer used by us, went on to our younger cousins. We each had a bicycle, but it was communicated to us that this one bike was to last through our childhood. I had my bike from age 7–14, when it was donated to a needy younger relative. My three sisters and I "recycled" our clothes. We convinced our mother to buy each one of us a popular "poor boy" sweater and skirt set in every pastel color. We mixed and match clothes to appear as if we had quite a sizable wardrobe.

Other recycling "traditions" included the obligatory covering of all textbooks with paper grocery bags, which must be completed "yesterday." There was once a widespread bag shortage panic. My mother had not yet gone grocery shopping that week. This was serious business, as failure to cover textbooks was a crime punishable by "staying after school."

The account above gives only a glimpse into the baby boomer cultural experience. However, the legacy passed on is a testament to the power of a generation to drive change and shape the future. Today, baby boomers make up approximately one fifth of the U.S. population. By 2041, it is projected to include one tenth. Our children and grandchildren now comprise a significant part of the workforce. But the effects of this population's presence in meeting the challenges of a generation for three quarters of a century resonates today.

References

Albaqawi, H., Butcon, V., Albagawi, B., Dayrit R. & Petelyne, P. (2021). Holistic nursing care among operating room nurses: Strengthening the standard of practice in Saudi Arabia. *Belitung Nursing Journal, 7*(1), 8–14.

Algoso, M., Ramjan, L., East, L., & Peters, K. (2024). Teaching and learning the art of nursing through aged care work experience. *Teaching & Learning in Nursing*, *19*(1), e89–e95.

Ambushe, S. A., Awoke, N., Demissie, B. W., & Tekalign, T. (2023). Holistic nursing care practice and associated factors among nurses in public hospitals of Wolaita zone, South Ethiopia. *BMC Nursing, 22*(1), 390. https://doi.org/10.1186/s12912-023-01517-0

Cai, D., He, W., & Klug, D. (2021). Cultural competence among nurses and its influencing factors: A cross-sectional study. *Nursing and Health Sciences, 23*, 411–418. https://doi.org/ https://doi.org/10.1111/nhs.12821

Červený, M., Kratochvílová, I., Hellerová, V., & Tóthová, V. (2022). Methods of increasing cultural competence in nurses working in clinical practice: A scoping review of literature 2011–2021. *Frontiers in Psychology, 13*, 936181. https://doi.org/10.3389/fpsyg.2022.936181

Douglas, M. K., Pierce, J. U., Rosenkoetter, M., Pacquiao, D., Callister, L. C., Hattar-Pollara, M., Lauderdale, J., Milstead, J., Nardi, D., & Purnell, L. (2011). Standards of practice for culturally competent nursing care. *Journal of Transcultural Nursing, 22*(4), 317–333. https://doi.org/10.1177/1043659611412965

Galanti, G. A. (2014). *Caring for patients from different cultures* (5th ed.). University of Pennsylvania Press

George, A. S. (2025). The baby boomers—a retrospective and prospective look at their enduring societal influence. *Partners Universal International Research Journal, 04*(01), 1–11. https://doi.org/10.5281/zenodo.15085643

Grewal, U. S., Abduljabar, H., & Sulaiman, K. (2021). Cultural competency in graduate medical education: A necessity for the minimization of disparities in healthcare. *EClinicalMedicine, 35*, 100837. https://doi.org/10.1016/j.eclinm.2021.100837

Kaihlanen, A., Hietapakka, L., & Heponiemi, T. (2019). Increasing cultural awareness: Qualitative study of nurses' perceptions about cultural competence training. *BMC Nursing,18*, 38. https://doi.org/10.1186/s12912-019-0363-x

Leininger, M. (1991). *Culture care diversity and universality: A theory of nursing.* National League for Nursing.

Lu, C., & Wan, C. (2018). Cultural self-awareness as awareness of culture's influence on the self: Implications for cultural identification and well-being. *Personality and Social Psychology Bulletin, 44*(6), 823–837. https://doi.org/10.1177/0146167217752117

Mager, N. D., & Moore, T. S. (2020). Healthy People 2030: Roadmap for public health for the next decade. *American Journal of Pharmaceutical Education, 84*(11), 8462. https://doi.org/10.5688/ajpe8462

Mande, J., & Flaherty, G. (2023). Supplemental nutrition assistance program as a health intervention. *Current Opinion in Pediatrics, 35*(1), 33–38. https://doi.org/10.1097/MOP.00000000000

McFarland, M. R., & Wehbe-Alamah, H. B. (2019). Leininger's theory of culture care diversity and universality: An overview with a historical retrospective and a view toward the future. *Journal of Transcultural Nursing, 30*(6), 540–557. https://doi.org/10.1177/1043659619867134

Narayan, M. C., & Mallinson, R. K. (2022). Transcultural nurse views on culture-sensitive/patient-centered assessment and care planning: A descriptive study. *Journal of Transcultural Nursing, 33*(2), 150–160. https://doi.org/10.1177/10436596211046986

Office of Disease Prevention and Health Promotion. (n.d.). Social determinants of health. *Healthy People 2030*. U.S. Department of Health and Human Services. https://health.gov/healthypeople/objectives-and-data/social-determinants-health

Olshansky E. F. (2017). Social determinants of health: The role of nursing. *The American Journal of Nursing, 117*(12), 11. https://doi.org/10.1097/01.NAJ.0000527463.16094.39

Pronk, N. P., Kleinman, D. V., & Richmond, T. S. (2021). Healthy people 2030: Moving toward Equitable Health and well-being in the United States. *EClinicalMedicine, 33*, 100777. https://doi.org/10.1016/j.eclinm.2021.100777

Riley, E., Haggard-Duff, L., & Long, C. R. (2020). Using an online learning module to teach nursing students about food insecurity as a social determinant of health. *Teaching and Learning in Nursing, 15*(4), 241–244. https://doi.org/10.1016/j.teln.2020.04.007

Suárez-Orozco, C., & Suárez-Orozco, M. M. (2001). *Children of immigration.* Harvard University Press.

Valdez, A., Fontenot, J., Millan, A., & McMurray, P. (2023). Knowledge, skills, and attitudes about diversity, equity, and inclusion among nurse educators. *Teaching & Learning in Nursing, 18*(2), 308–316.

Williams, M., Dubree, M., & Schorn, M. (2025). Effective nurse diversity, equity, and inclusion programs: A guide for health care institutions. *Nurse Leader, 0(0)* 1–9. 1541-4612/2025 https://doi.org/10.1016/j.mnl.2024.12.011

World Health Organization. (2022). *Constitution of the World Health Organization.* https://www.who.int/about/governance/constitution

■ CHAPTER 12

Informatics Literacy

Strengthening Informatics and Health Information Literacy

Let us never consider ourselves finished nurses ... we must be learning all of our lives.

—Florence Nightingale

Social distancing restrictions challenged care provision during the COVID-19 pandemic. However, the use of informatics and telehealth technology accelerated significantly for providers and their patients. With access to remote patient care, providers recognized the associated benefits of this practice, including efficiency of treatment, reduced travel time, and a greater potential for patient compliance with care.

While this data-driven knowledge is essential for improving patient care, the process of acquiring and applying it can be daunting for health care professionals. For overburdened nurses, there is increased pressure to balance clinical responsibilities with the ongoing need for continuing education and professional development. Establishing informatics literacy as a nurse is a critical part of the profession, but it often demands significant time and effort, adding to the already high levels of stress that nurses face daily in their professional roles. Nurses may feel underprepared or overwhelmed by the technological demands of their role (Khalid et al., 2024). For some, embracing technology is challenging; for those entering the nursing profession who grew up with technology, it is an expansion of their current knowledge, experience, and expertise.

Growing use of information systems in the health care setting has significantly changed the daily workflow of nurses. The increased use of information systems, while critical for improving patient care and other hospital administrative processes, requires nurses and other staff members to develop a strong competence in informatics.

Kotter's Model of Change

Never doubt that a small group of thoughtful committed people can change the world, indeed it is the only thing that ever has

—Margaret Mead

As a complex and multifaceted phenomenon threaded through individuals' lives, adapting to change is difficult. The process of change is an inevitable issue in healthcare. Therefore, understanding the benefits of change for providers and patients is most likely to be successful when "changemakers" have the opportunity to influence modifications in care and treatment interventions. Kotter's (1996) Eight Step Change Model can help nurses and other health care professionals to overcome change, adopt new processes, and embrace advancing technology skills, in the provision of informed, current, and safe patient care.

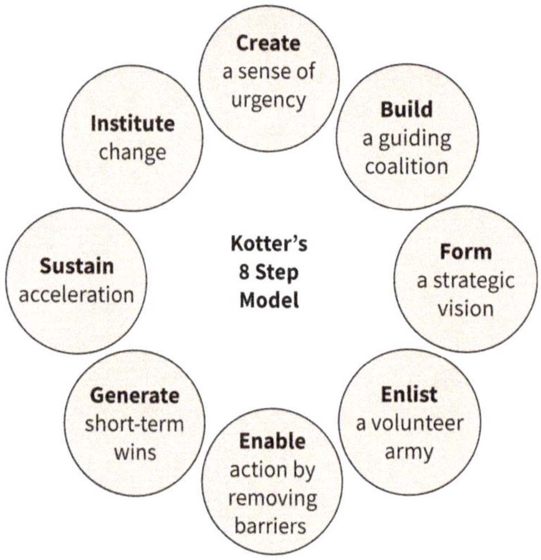

Figure 12.1 Kotter's Eight-Step Model of Organizational Change

Kotter's (1996) model consists of eight stages. **Step One** involves creating a climate for change by establishing a sense of urgency. Creating urgency is imperative because staff may resist change if unaware of an existing issue. A high level of motivation in the target audience is crucial for the change process to succeed. Therefore, people need to be convinced that the change is necessary now. This sense of urgency will propel them toward accepting and finally implementing the change.

With **Step Two**, guiding associations includes the creation of a team of capable and influential leaders from the organization. The team should be informed and goal-oriented in order to influence others to accept and champion the change. **Step Three** incorporates the development of a clear vision for the change. Team members collaborate to further refine goals toward achieving the change, while still focusing on the vision. In **Step Four**, the team approaches "target" people with "bold talk" of the vision and goals. The aim here is to gain people's support through straightforward, plain speech, ensuring adequate time for encouraging dialogue and fostering clear understanding of the proposed change (Kotter,1996).

The goal of **Step Five** lies in engaging others to act. Encouraging "buy in" while trouble shooting potential barriers to change (knowledge deficits, existing organizational structures, workers' skill sets) can empower staff to better understand how they "fit" into this change, and what role they might play in the changed environment. **Step Six** incorporates the creation of "short-term wins," a series of small steps to the larger, intended goal. Short-term wins aid in overcoming obstructions and can steer the change process toward long-term successes.

Step Seven involves sustaining the momentum by anticipating the possible return of disruptions while ensuring any obstacles do not deter the change process. In maintaining a focus on the vision and plan to move forward, this mindset inspires and empowers individuals to welcome the change. Finally, **Step Eight** incorporates the change into the culture. It becomes the standard, viewed as necessary and beneficial over the previous way of working. New employees see this change as part of the culture (Kotter, 1996).

Kotter's change management theory is a dynamic model that delineates the process of "leading" change. In particular, this model can be invaluable for health care leaders to alleviate staff stress, enhance the adjustment process, and embrace technology (Duphily, 2022).

Informatics Technology (IT) Education

For those entering nursing programs, incorporating technological advances and educational tools in active learning environments can significantly enhance the development of different skills, particularly in fields like nursing where information literacy is critical. By increasing engagement, personalizing learning experiences, and providing opportunities for collaboration, these tools help students develop confidence in their IT abilities and become better prepared for real-world challenges. The use of these resources not only alleviates stress but also fosters competence, leading to greater success in both academic and professional settings (Kaihlanen et al., 2021). For both entry-level and returning nursing students, active learning plays a pivotal role in enhancing student success, particularly in contexts such as academic and clinical settings, where developing information literacy is essential.

Active learning can be applied to increase student engagement. This can be seen in the use of interactive quizzes, discussion boards, forums, and other methods that allow instructors to adjust content based on the learner's needs. These tools increase the access to resources and offer more opportunity for feedback, as well as provides students with more power over their learning, thus creating environments that allow students to be actively involved in their education (Khalid et al., 2024). The assertions made by Khalid et al. (2024) reinforce experiences where simulated and computerized clinical practice training were used to increase nurses' engagement and understanding. The use of technology-based learning is significantly helpful during team building activities and skills development day in the emergency setting as this can reinforce skills that nurses use on everyday, real-life patient encounters.

Telehealth

Telehealth uses electronic information and telecommunications technology to cultivate remote clinical healthcare, improve health-related education and public health needs, and support health administration (Duphily, 2022). This technology enables increased access to care for those with geographic, cultural, physical, social, or financial barriers.

Telehealth nursing quality is described as a multidimensional concept that encompasses attributes such as empathy, assurance, and reliability (Duphily, 2022). Telehealth nurses must possess informatics skills in order to successfully provide virtual care, access patient information, and collaborate with patients, family, and other health care members.

In 2018, a pilot study was conducted to review and assess the quality of care delivered by nurses within a telehealth organization. Bashir and Bastola (2018) reported that nurses and patients had positive experiences with this form of care delivery. The authors concluded that telehealth improved interprofessional communication, safety, and patient quality of life, and allowed clinicians to customize patient care quickly and effectively.

Telehealth promises valuable potential for health care delivery by providing evidence-based, efficient, and cost-effective care, while also enhancing education and timely communication between health care providers and patients (Davis et al., 2020). By using telehealth, providers can employ real-time assessment, remote monitoring, and virtual follow-ups that enable providers to administer timely interventions and maintain continuity of care. Telehealth can also enhance communication between patients and nurses and foster better adherence to treatment plans, in turn increasing compliance and overall patient outcomes.

The Use of "Wearables"

Nurses comprise a major proportion of direct patient care hours. Patient acuity and complexity of care have escalated significantly, with factors such as understaffing of nurses and an aging patient population leading to increased workloads and mounting stress. Ultimately, these demands pose major risks to nurses' physical and mental health, quality of life, role satisfaction, and job retention. Those nurses remaining on understaffed units face an increasing burden with overextended workloads, which negatively impacts the quality of patient care and outcomes (Buchholz, 2023).

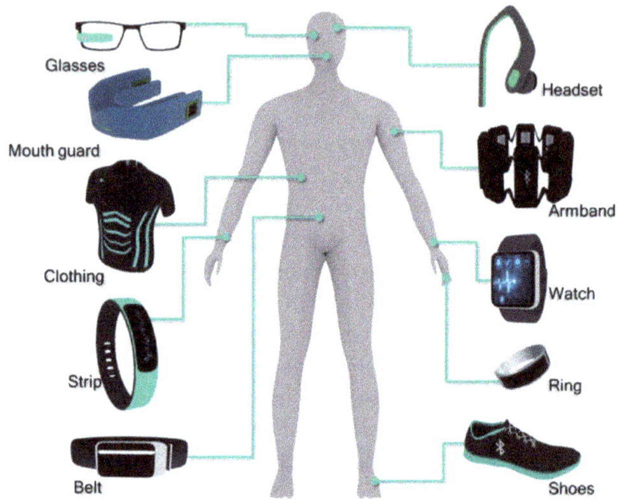

Figure 12.2 Wearables

Wearable devices may be the answer. Their popularity is growing among the general public. Small, noninvasive electronic devices attached to clothes, worn as a device attached to the body or directly to the skin (Fitbit tracker, Apple Watch), wearables are embedded with sensors and wireless mobility. The data generated in the use of wearables could prove valuable in improving the delivery of care for patients in both outpatient and inpatient settings (Buchholz, 2023).

Virtual care in nursing can help with data collection, patient admission and discharge, patient education, and family education. With wearable technology for patients, nurses can monitor vital signs and patient status, freeing up staff so they can spend time attending to other responsibilities. Wearables also have the potential to help with hospital home care, because patients can continue wearing the technology that will keep monitoring their progress (Kang et al., 2022).

The Nursing Informatics Specialist (NIS)

Efficiency counts when nurses provide patient care. It begins with the ability to access accurate patient health information. Both electronic health records (EHR) and electronic medical records (EMR) afford health care providers the ability to quickly enter and review accurate and secure patient health information. As part of a collaborative team of health care providers, nurses recognize the value and need of information necessary in order to provide efficient, informed, and effective clinical care to their patients. NI serves to bridge the gap between clinical and technological aspects of patient care. The NIS serves the dual role of innovative technology advocate and mentor, while focusing on patient safety and privacy (American Nurses Association [ANA], 2022).

The ANA (2022) describes informatics as the integration of nursing science, computer science, and information science to manage and communicate data, information, knowledge, and wisdom in nursing practice. This data approach to patient care enhances the clinical experience for health care providers and patients.

Individuals interested in a NIS position must possess a minimum of a bachelor of science in nursing (BSN). Essential skills include clinical experience and an understanding of the information needs of a health care setting; proficiency in EHRs and data analytics; an ability to adapt to emerging, dynamic technology; and project management skills related to system implementation, improvements, troubleshooting, and upgrades.

In the education of and collaboration with individuals from different departments in the hospital organization, strong communication skills with interdisciplinary teams regarding technology use are mandatory for NIS candidates. As an advocate for nursing ethics and patient safety and privacy, the NIS's role contributes a nursing voice to the IT team and plays a major role in contributing to the adoption of new processes and programs (Duphily, 2022).

The NIS encourages informatics literacy for both providers and patients. Employing nursing focused, ethical perspectives, the NIS maintains the quality and safety of care through efforts (data analysis, visualization, and presentation skills) to ensure positive patient outcomes and nursing staff satisfaction (Nelson & Parker, 2019).

As a visionary, advocate, and voice for nurses and patients, the NIS plays a vital role in linking technology and data to transform health care delivery, enhance patient outcomes, and advance the nursing profession. This nursing role bridges a health care organization's systems, nursing staff, and providers, including nurse practitioners and certified nurse midwives. Incorporating the field of informatics into the discipline nursing offers valuable input into how technological systems should be designed and implemented from a nursing perspective.

Reflective Questions

1. How has the introduction of EHR affected nursing workflow, communication, and patient outcomes in acute care settings?
2. Do you feel that telehealth technology influences health care access, especially in rural and underserved communities?
3. How do wearable health devices impact a person's health self-management?
4. Do you feel that home remote monitoring technology impacts health care quality? Why?

Kotter's Model of Change

Consider a change you would like to make in your organization.

1. What resources will you identify?
2. What are the time considerations for change to be implemented?
3. What individuals will you involve in your plan for change?
4. Will the change

- improve the outcomes you had hoped for,
- help you more accurately identify areas for improvement,
- increase safety and efficiency in your workplace, or
- resolve previous barriers?

Scenario

The Role of the Nurse Informatics Specialist

Ryan has been a registered nurse for 12 years. Four years ago, he received an advanced nursing degree in nursing informatics and has been employed since as one of three NIS within a large metropolitan teaching hospital. In the ongoing role of ensuring the integrity and security of health care data, Ryan and his colleagues work to enhance the use of EHRs, modify workflows, and recognize opportunities for process improvement.

As a regional nursing informaticist, Ryan's role requires travel to two other states, to hospitals within a wide-ranging health care organization. Ryan brings his cell phone and laptop computer to these sites. When he is working from home, he uses several electronic devices: cell phone, desktop computer, and laptop. Occasionally he must log into the computer system to see patient's information in order to troubleshoot problems within the electronic medical record.

Questions

1. What potential security risks are posed for Ryan outside of the hospital setting, with both travel and working from home?
2. What actions can Ryan take to stay safe online (i.e., password choices; two-factor identification, antivirus software)?
3. How can Ryan protect his cell phone, and desktop, and laptop computers from cybercriminals?
4. Have you observed the introduction of a new computer system in your workplace?
5. What benefits of health technology have you seen or experienced? Disadvantages noted?

Food for Thought

Closing the Education to Practice Gap Through Informatics

The American Recovery and Reinvestment Act of 2009, signed by President Obama, included $19.2 billion in provisions for health care information technology. The act authorized the Centers for Medicare and Medicaid Services to provide reimbursement incentives for providers who are successful in becoming meaningful users of EHRs (Alexandre & Glazer, 2009).

Regis College, in Weston, Massachusetts, addressed the demands of education and professional development of health professionals by developing a program that links to the institution's strategic goal of expanding experiential learning opportunities. The program employs a case study based method in the classroom. Faculty work with students to design field experiences most appropriate to meet their professional goals.

One such experiential assignment is highlighted next with this DNP student's journal entry for an informatics technology project, guided by educator and IT specialist Mark Sugrue:

Today, the CIO from the hospital visited the college with wonderful news regarding a collaborative project first proposed by this writer as part of a class assignment in the Regis Informatics course this fall, taught by Mark Sugrue. The plan consists of a partnership between the local community college and hospital organization to establish a "mock-up" hospital computer system, to be housed at the community college campus. Both institutions are located across the street from one another.

This program would introduce the community college's nursing students to the hospital's electronic documentation system right here on the college campus. This preclinical orientation would provide hands on computer instruction at the college and practice in a stress-free classroom, with sufficient time for learning, comfortable space, and guidance from experienced users. Hospital staff will collaborate with nursing faculty, many of whom work at the hospital on a part-time basis, to streamline, troubleshoot, and complete the clinical orientation process on site. The goal here is to reduce orientation stress.

Historically, it was noted to be difficult to accommodate computer orientation for the many nursing students entering this hospital's clinical setting. This strategy helps to meet the objective of integrating informatics into the curriculum and enhances professional growth from student to clinician.

This initiative provides an example of how the DNP program at Regis fosters returning students' goal to make each graduate course "count." It has helped this writer personally and professionally in a new leadership career. Moreover, the Capstone Project illustrates the importance of investment by organizations in guiding the next generation of nurses, with their collaborative efforts in paving the way.

References

Alexandre, C., & Glazer, G., (2009, June 22). Legislative: The American Recovery and Reinvestment Act of 2009: What's in it for nursing? *OJIN: The Online Journal of Issues in Nursing, 14* (3), 1–2. https://doi.org/10.3912/OJIN.Vol14No03LegCol01

American Nurses Association. (2022). *Nursing Informatics: Scope and standards of practice* (3rd ed.).

Bashir, A., & Bastola, D. R. (2018). Perspectives of nurses toward telehealth efficacy and quality of health care: Pilot study. *JMIR Medical Informatics*, *6*(2). https://doi.org/10.2196/medinform.9080

Buchholz, S. W., Mowbray, F. I., Allman, G., Verboncoeur, J. P., Beam, L., & Small, L. (2023). Wearable devices and nurses' health: Protocol for an integrative review. *JMIR Research Protocols*, *12*, e48178. https://doi.org/10.2196/48178

Davis, S. M., Jones, A., Jaynes, M. E., Woodrum, K. N., Canaday, M., Allen, L., & Mallow, J. A. (2020). Designing a multifaceted telehealth intervention for a rural population using a model for developing complex interventions in nursing. *BMC Nursing*, *19*(1), 1–9. https://doi-org.fitchburgstate.idm.oclc.org/10.1186/s12912-020-0400-9

Duphily, N. (2022). *Moving from your associate to your baccalaureate nursing degree* (1st ed.). Cognella Academic Publishing.

Kaihlanen, A.-M., Gluschkoff, K., Laukka, E., & Heponiemi, T. (2021). The information system stress, informatics competence, and well-being of newly graduated and experienced nurses: A cross-sectional study. *BMC Health Services Research*, *21*(1), 1–8.

Kang, H. S., & Exworthy, M. (2022). Wearing the future: Wearables to empower users to take greater responsibility for their health and care: Scoping review. *JMIR mHealth and uHealth*, *10*(7), e35684. https://doi.org/10.2196/35684

Khalid, N., Zapparrata, N., & Phillips, B. C. (2024). Theoretical underpinnings of technology-based interactive instruction. *Teaching & Learning in Nursing*, *19*(1), e145–e149. https://doi-org.fitchburgstate.idm.oclc.org/10.1016/j.teln.2023.10.004

Kotter, J. P. (1996). *Leading change*. Harvard Business School Press.

Nelson, T. L., & Parker, C. D. (2019). Nursing informatics: The EHR and beyond. *American Nurse Today*, *14*(3), 1–3.

Figure Credits

Fig. 12.1: P. Srinivas Subbarao and Puneet Kumar, "Kotter's Eight-Step Model of Organizational Change," *Organizational Leadership and Change Management*, p. 16. Copyright © 2021 by Paramount Publishing House.

Fig. 12.2: Kyeonghye Guk et al., "Evolution of Wearable Devices with Real-Time Disease Monitoring for Personalized Healthcare," *Nanometals*, vol. 9, no. 6, p. 3, MDPI. Copyright © 2019 by Kyeonghye Guk et al. (CC BY 4.0) at https://www.mdpi.com/2079-4991/9/6/813.

■ CHAPTER 13

Quality Improvement

Quality Improvement and Patient-Centered Care

Our greatest weakness lies in giving up. The most certain way to succeed is always to try just one more time.

—Thomas Edison

Introduction

Quality improvement (QI) in nursing is defined as a strategic and systematic approach to evaluating health care services and nursing practices to improve patient care and outcomes. At a time when the needs of patients are becoming more complex, it has never been more important to focus on QI in nursing. In order to maintain continuous QI, nurses must identify issues in need of change and implement improvement strategies. Patient-centered care rests at the heart of QI in nursing. Understanding the holistic needs and preferences of patients plays a central role in improving outcomes, as providers strive for quality, inclusive care to earn the trust of the patients they serve.

Patient-centered care is an essential key to improving patient satisfaction ratings and achieving better overall outcomes. In prioritizing the needs of patients, nurses demonstrate an awareness of their concerns, their cultural values, and their general comfort level. In addition to prioritizing the physical health of their patients, nurses must also consider their patients' emotional health. By being aware of the needs of patients and balancing their emotional and physical health concerns, nurses can better advocate for their patients as they work with providers to develop a personalized treatment plan.

The Quality Improvement Model

The QI model consists of four steps: identifying, analyzing, planning, and implementing/testing (Dolansky et al., 2024):

- **Identifying the problem**. Before nurses and health care leaders can begin collaborating to make improvements, they must first identify challenges and shortcomings within their systems. Problems can be identified by evaluating patient data, observing patient care practices within a facility, or conducting a survey to gauge the pulse of the community being served.
- **Gathering accurate and relevant data**. Once a problem has been identified, nurses and health care administrators should work together to collect data from the patient population to further explore how the problem can be addressed. Nurse informatics plays a vital role in QI.

- **Developing an intervention to solve the problem**. After data has been collected and analyzed, nurses can work to create targeted interventions that address the specific problem that exists.
- **Analyze the intervention's results**. Data collection efforts should continue even once the intervention has been implemented because evaluation and assessment are key parts of QI. It is important to ensure the intervention is working, as adjustments can be made accordingly.

The Plan-Do-Study-Act (PDSA) Cycle

Nurses and other providers have developed specific strategies to streamline the process of identifying areas for improvement and create targeted interventions that will lead to lasting results. One such strategy is the PDSA cycle (McNeil & Nevin, 2009), a systematic series of steps to identify a patient, process, or system. The PDSA cycle is particularly valuable because it relies heavily on data collection and analysis to verify that a QI intervention works as intended. It can be used for interventions small in scope, making it one of the most practical QI tools. As a practical and easy-to-use framework, the PDSA cycle can assist nurses to implement QI projects. Additionally, it gives nurses the ability to track the results of their interventions to adopt systematic and aligned behaviors.

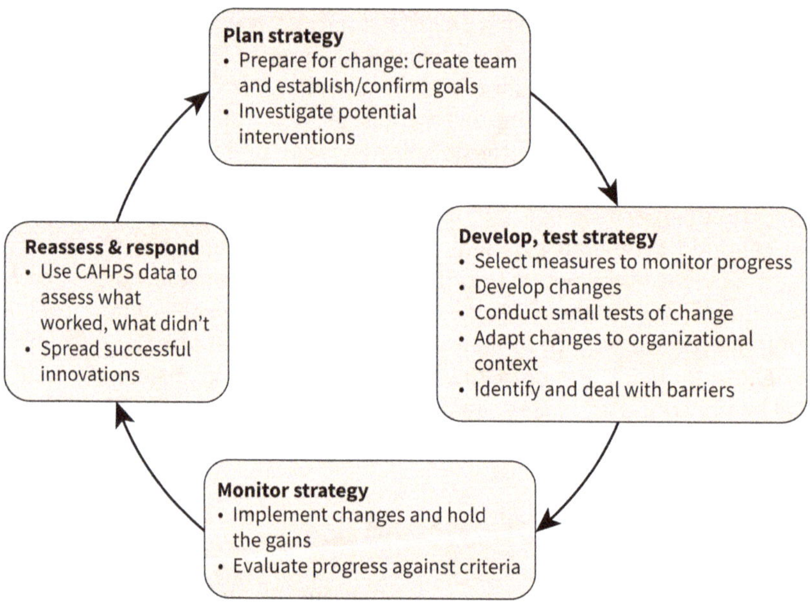

Figure 13.1 The Plan-Do-Study-Act Cycle

QI and Root Cause Analysis (RCA)

RCA is a strategic process for nurses that focuses on QI in the profession. When patients experience unexpected, serious adverse outcomes, RCA aids in analysis of the situation. RCA assists providers to examine, recognize, and strategize ways to prevent issues from recurring (Duphily, 2022).

RCA requires health care professionals to follow specific protocols in collecting relevant data to better understand the patient experience. In certain instances, patient and participant interviews are recorded to document the events as they occur. RCA involves analysis of the events that occurred in order to identify the errors that led to the negative outcome and determine the root cause of the event, why they occurred in the first place, and what actions need to be taken to prevent similar situations from happening in the future.

QI and Lewin's Change Theory

If you want to truly understand something, try to change it.

—Kurt Lewin

QI involves changing and evolving practices that may instigate challenges. Even if the change is beneficial, staff uncertainty with the potential change may occur. Lewin's (1951) change management theory offers a strategic approach that can assist nurses in planning, implementing, and evaluating the proposed change (Payne, 2013).

Kurt Lewin's change theory can be utilized in healthcare to help staff adjust to change to efficiently adopt and maintain the development. Lewin's model represents a dynamic balance of forces working in opposing directions to create a "push-pull" effect as an individual navigates through the process of change (Duphily, 2022). These energies include driving forces, restraining forces, and equilibrium. Restraining forces are those life experiences that oppose change (Duphily, 2022). In a study involving organizational commitment to implementing the electronic health record technology, restraining forces would include inadequate training, unsupportive management, staff resistance, reluctance to learn something new, insufficient financial resources, negative organizational culture, high costs, and privacy concerns (Payne, 2013). Forces that inspire change, driving forces, would include the desire to improve the documentation, the belief that electronic documentation facilitates access to accurate and comprehensive clinical information, adequate training, and positive attitudes, the desire to expand personal knowledge, sufficient financial resources, and positive organizational culture (Payne, 2013). Equilibrium occurs when forces are equal. When this happens, a change in driving or restraining forces must occur to steer individuals in the desired direction.

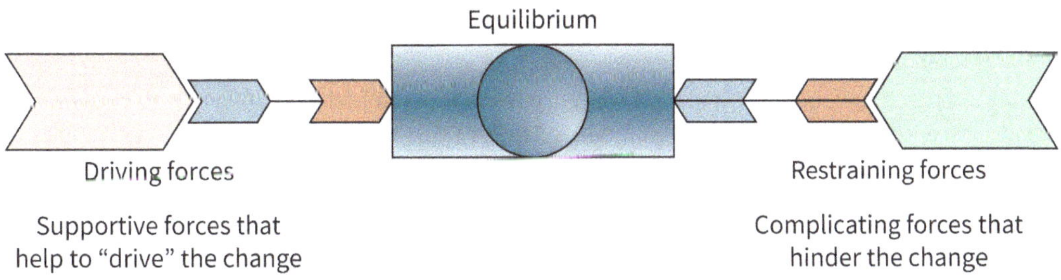

Figure 13.2 Force Field Analysis

Benefits of Quality Improvement

By recognizing their role in the QI process, nurses can better advocate for patients by developing informed interventions that lead to positive changes in the workplace setting. When nurses play an active role in QI projects, the outcomes are significantly better. Nurses at all levels have the opportunity and ability to advocate for their patients and take on leadership roles within QI projects. By proactively working to participate in QI initiatives, nurses can advocate for better patient care standards while also offering input as to the best way to improve patient outcomes at their health care facility. The nurses who become involved in QI initiatives find it a rewarding process, one in which they can see the direct results of their efforts.

QI in nursing is a collaborative effort, and all members of the care team should work together to identify areas for improvement and develop strategic solutions. Engaging the entire nursing team in QI efforts not only promotes collaboration in the health care landscape but also leads to more comprehensive and successful initiatives.

Nurse leaders can involve nursing team members in QI initiatives through transparent and frequent communication regarding the importance of quality improvement in the profession. Inspiring nursing team members to become involved in QI efforts can be accomplished through hosting regular QI meetings throughout all shifts, so that all team members can attend and participate. Finally, highlighting the contributions of others and recognizing them for their achievements inspires "buy in" from staff, to investigate and learn more about the benefits of QI initiatives.

Reflective Questions

1. If you were seeking to "improve the quality" of an area in your life (personally, professionally, workplace setting), where would you begin?
2. What areas would you want to focus on for improvement?
3. What are your goals? Specific actions toward these goals?
4. Who will be affected, and how?
5. Would you include others to help manage the project?
6. What resources and timeline would you need?
7. What are possible barriers, and how might you resolve them?
8. How would you measure success of your QI plan?

Scenario

Creating a Quality Improvement Program to Reduce Patient Falls

A major objective for health care delivery systems is in improving the patient experience. Health care administrators face significant challenges in their objective to align changes in behavior and practices across multiple levels and areas of the organization. It is incumbent upon health care leaders to take advantage of the established principles of, and approaches to, QI.

McHugh General Hospital has identified a significant rise in patient falls on one of their medical units. Recognizing the gravity of this threat to patient safety, hospital administration convened a meeting to strategize interventions for resolution of this problem. A QI project was created, beginning with the selection of a "Hospital Success Team." This group was composed of a "microsystem" of invested individuals from nursing, medicine, physical therapy, nursing management, and hospital administration. "Microsystems" are multiple small units of caregivers, administrators, and other staff who produce the "products" of healthcare; specifically, those individuals who deliver care and services (Likosky, 2014).

The aim of this QI project was "harm minimization." Together, the team identified goals for the project: improved communication among care providers, patient safety through adequate staffing, and dissemination and incorporation of current evidence related to "falls awareness," to inform best practices in patient-centered care.

"Falls" content focused on a "Topic of the Week." The "Hospital Success Team" members chose key themes and content related to the concept of falls. Team members then disseminated the information via email each week to staff within their discipline, with direct links to key content relating to the particular week's theme. Weekly focus topics contributed both knowledge for new staff and a refresher for "veterans." Feedback was encouraged; staff could request further information, add information from their own research on falls, ask questions, or share experiences that they felt would benefit others in the group. Additionally, positive messages about improvement of falls or responses by the team during the week were included.

Staff surveys following the first month of the QI project's initiation were positive. Staff revealed that in particular, the team's feedback to their suggestions made them "feel heard." They cited improvement in the timing and ease of access of information conveyed. Staff believed that the "give-and-take" feedback felt more personal and was acknowledged and respected through this project's method of communication. Previously, progress with projects was unclear. Evidence was often presented "as an afterthought" along with other agenda items during monthly unit meetings. In this situation, the frequent updates and announcements acknowledging progress toward the goal were meaningful, supportive, and motivating.

Questions

1. What evidence would you expect to see if the QI falls reduction project was successful?
2. How would the team use the PDSA cycle in their fall prevention plan?
3. What other communication techniques could be used to convey educational materials to interdisciplinary staff?
4. What additional interventions would foster achieving the expected outcome?
5. Have you participated in QI projects? If so, what was your role? What was the experience like for you?

Food for Thought

Inspiring Quality Improvement in Nursing: A Clinical Practice Guideline Project

More than ever, health care organizations seek nursing graduates, empowered through education, who are able to critique existing practices and initiate evidence-based changes, resulting in better patient outcomes. This ability is a vital part of a nursing philosophy, which focuses on evidence-based QI. Evidence-based practice is a problem-solving approach that incorporates the thorough use of up-to-date, quality data in decisions regarding patient care. It involves a systematic search for the most relevant evidence, as well as critical appraisal of this evidence to answer a clinical question (Fineout-Overholt et al., 2010; Melnyk & Fineout-Overholt, 2011).

Empowered with this knowledge, junior baccalaureate nursing faculty at university created an interactive project to involve students in the entire evidence-based practice (EBP) process, with the intent of increasing their understanding and value of its impact on nursing quality. The undergraduate nursing faculty came together to examine the current course's teaching and evaluation strategies for the class *Evidence-Based Practice in Nursing.* Upon review of various texts, as well as the course curriculum and outline, it was discovered that content concentrated on competencies in research activities rather than a focus on the importance of finding current evidence as a necessary tool for best practice. Faculty discussion and student feedback from prior course evaluations revealed that content of this course should integrate evidence-based strategies related to clinical practice.

Expectations for new nursing graduates require EBP expertise for QI in the present and future settings of complex care delivery systems. Students now must demonstrate experience navigating diverse information technology systems, as well as possess technical skill competencies for timely retrieval of current, relevant information necessary for the multifaceted care of patients (IOM, 2010).With the goal of employing an interactive approach in teaching an evidence-based undergraduate nursing course, as well as aligning the curriculum to reflect the current AACN Essentials, the *Evidence-Based Practice in Nursing* course description was revised: "This course will introduce the student to the implementation of evidence-based learning strategies. By the end of this semester, the student will be able to identify a question, examine and appraise current literature, and evaluate practice protocols" in furthering QI. Also, course outcomes were modified to reflect the following skills acquisition by nursing students:

Prior to the start of the semester, *Evidence-Based Practice in Nursing* course faculty met with nursing educators from the medical center where the university nursing students complete their clinical experience. Both groups discussed ways to foster the use of current evidence in the clinical setting, for students, novices, and veteran nurses. The idea for a collaborative strategy used to demonstrate the importance of actively linking evidence to practice in nursing education was generated. As part of an interactive, collaborative component to the *Evidence-Based Practice in Nursing* course, students selected specific clinical practice guidelines (CPGs) in need of current review, as recommended by medical center nursing staff educators. Nursing student competencies for EBP, national health care improvement priorities, evidence rating systems, and a model of knowledge transformation for EBP provided the impetus for the establishment of such a venture. Students examining the CPGs would appraise the evidence supporting the recommendation for change in health care practice and compare the recommendation to actual practice. The idea for a future forum during which students could exhibit their work to staff nurses (poster presentations) was considered, and a preliminary plan was created.

CPGs reviewed included catheter associated urinary tract infections (CAUTI), central line associated bloodstream infections (CLABSI), flushing of central lines, suicide prevention, hourly rounding to enhance fall prevention, blind insertion versus X-ray confirmation for enteral tube feeding, rapid response, pediatric early warning system (PEWS), breastfeeding and neonatal abstinence syndrome (NAS), workplace violence, family presence during invasive procedures/resuscitation, handoffs/bedside reporting, and adolescent suicide prevention: a community approach.

Interactive class dialogue served to measure student understanding of the concepts surrounding critical appraisal of evidence. Group work gave students the opportunity to discuss the content of EBP in a less threatening atmosphere, a classroom of their peers. During discussions, students were engaged in helping, listening to, and learning from each other. In evaluation of this activity, students credited lecture, group work, and interactive discussion at each step of the article appraisal as efficient, effective ways of learning to evaluate a scientific article.

The CPG project, as part of the *Evidence-Based Practice in Nursing* course, culminated in formal oral and power point presentations by each group at the end of the semester. Students were also invited to present their work as poster presentations in both Shared Leadership Day at the Medical Center and the Annual Student Research Day at the University. Working collaboratively on this project provided an opportunity for students to discuss the significance, influence, and strength of the evidence supporting the recommendation to change health care practice.

It is critical that student nurses know when and how to practice using evidence-based research. As students, if they achieve the skills needed to ask sound research questions, acquire evidence-based answers to their questions, and interpret their findings into practice, they will thrive in the profession. Through this process, students in the EBP class acknowledged the value of examining current, relevant literature. They developed an appreciation for the university's library staff and the library's database resources, as well as the contributions of both nursing and multidisciplinary research for quality patient care. From this experience, students' recommendations included: identification of hospital and nursing administration stakeholders in order to garner full support and encouragement in bringing the CPG project's recommendations to fruition, frequent interdisciplinary communication to keep the health care team abreast of updates and changes, and ongoing staff in-services to focus on compliance with current guideline recommendations.

Students gained skills in reviewing evidence, classifying references, and applying data to recommend improvements in health care practices. The project assisted students in recognizing the full process of change, from knowledge development to application in practice improvements. Collaborative experiential activities within student groups stimulated critical thinking and dialogue. Small group meetings held during the instructor's scheduled office hours were beneficial in identifying potential gaps in knowledge during important intervals and due dates in student work progression. Moreover, student groups acquired knowledge and experience related to professional roles through poster presentations, peer review, and feedback. Expectations regarding professional dress and comportment conveyed the significance of formal collegial atmosphere, research, requirements for poster presentations, and the role of peer review.

Although EBP can be taught formally in a lecture format, providing students with active learning assignments can reinforce these skills and fortify learning. Nursing students need to be actively involved in the scholarship of EBP in order to develop a systematic way of thinking through clinical situations to provide optimal patient care. If these skills are developed early on in their education and incorporated, practiced, and refined through each course in the nursing curriculum, it becomes "second nature" to them, leading ultimately to a lifelong nursing career and philosophy that bases everyday practice on evidence.

References

Dolansky, M. A., Horvat Davey, C., & Moore, S. M. (2024). Research and practice in quality improvement and implementation science: The synergy for change model. *Journal of Nursing Care Quality*, *39*(3), 199–205. https://doi.org/10.1097/NCQ.0000000000000760

Duphily, N. (2022). *Moving from your associate to your baccalaureate nursing degree* (1st ed.). Cognella Academic Publishing.

Fineout-Overholt, E., Melnyk, B., Stillwell, S. & Williamson, K. (2010). Evidence-based practice step by step: Critical appraisal of the evidence: Part I. *American Journal of Nursing*, *110* (7), 47–52. https://doi.org/10.1097/01.NAJ.0000383935.22721.9c

Institute of Medicine. (2010). *The future of nursing: Leading change, advancing health*. National Academies Press.

Lewin, K. (1951). *Field theory in social science*. Harper.

Likosky, D. S. (2014). Clinical microsystems: A critical framework for crossing the quality chasm. *The Journal of Extra-Corporeal Technology*, *46*(1), 33–37.

McNeil, M. M., & Nevin, A. I. (2009), Communication: The key to effective leadership. *Journal of Educational Administration*, *47*(5), 684–687. https://doi.org/10.1108/09578230910981161

Melnyk, B., & Fineholt-Overholt, E. (2011). *Evidence-based practice in nursing and healthcare: A guide for best practice* (2nd ed.). Lippincott.

Payne, S. (2013). The implementation of electronic clinical documentation using Lewin's change management theory. *Canadian Journal of Nursing Informatics, 8* (2), 1–9.

Figure Credits

Fig. 13.1: Susan Edgman-Levitan et al., "Understanding and Implementing the Improvement Cycle," *The CAHPS Ambulatory Care Improvement Guide: Practical Strategies for Improving Patient Experience*, p. 29, https://www.ahrq.gov/sites/default/files/wysiwyg/cahps/quality-improvement/improvement-guide/cahps-ambulatory-care-guide-full.pdf. Copyright © 2017 by Yale School of Public Health. Reprinted with permission.

Fig. 13.2: June Kaminski, "The Change Process and Lewin's Theory," *Nursing Curriculum for Supporting Change*, https://www.nursing-informatics.com/N4111/LA1.html. Copyright © by Nursing Informatics Learning Center.

CHAPTER 14

Just the Beginning

Now this is not the end. It is not even the beginning of the end. But it is, perhaps, the end of the beginning.

—Winston Churchill

This final chapter might lead the reader to believe there is an ultimate "conclusion" or end to the current situation in nursing. In actuality, it is just the beginning. The intent of this book hopefully inspires and motivates the reader to participate in the creation of something new and exciting. Churchill's statement encourages optimism in fostering the profession's potential for positive growth and change rather than uncertainty and doubt. He challenges us to view endings as opportunities for new beginnings, informed by resilience and open-minded perspectives.

Nursing is a career of lifelong learning. In order to make a significant contribution to the advancement of nursing, long-term growth, and continual change, investing in the future is crucial. This is accomplished by staying informed, aware, and passionate. Passing on expertise and knowledge to the next generation of nursing professionals can actually help nurses to learn more through questions and explaining procedures and processes. The more nurses discuss the passion in their work, the more they strengthen their own knowledge on the subject matter. In conversations with mentees, mentors gain new perspectives from their questions, their educational background as well as their own experiences.

For experienced or "veteran" nurses, sharing years of experience in the profession and explaining the rationales behind interventions help shape the minds of future nursing leaders. Nurses have the power to make influential impacts on the nursing profession through continued education, networking opportunities, being politically active in nursing organizations, and finding a nursing community they can depend on for support and as a source of reliable information. Regardless of the detail or size of the contribution, sharing knowledge leads to advances in the profession.

Professional Development and Continuing Education

Enrollment in online continuing education courses, attending conferences, membership in a professional organization, and subscriptions to nursing journals offer a variety of ways to stay abreast of the dynamic nature of the discipline. Professional associations keep nurses informed on trending news, issues, and topics so all members of the organization are made aware of new research generated. Access to reliable sources enables nurses to apply evidence to practice, which ultimately propels the profession forward.

Attending events and conferences gives nurses the opportunity to obtain new knowledge and information and meet other nursing professionals outside of the workplace. Influencers in the profession come together, share their expertise on a subject, educate other professionals on a new process or procedure, and build networks. Exchanging ideas among professionals fosters knowledge and growth.

Memberships in nursing associations link nursing professionals who share the same passion for learning. This association fosters community and assists nurses to remain current in advances within their particular specialty in the nursing field. Moreover, networking globally with others who may have differing views on specific topics broadens perspectives and creates further discussion and exploration. Additionally, being a part of a nursing "community" helps prevent burnout. From the experiences many have shared during the COVID-19 pandemic, the fellowship of a support group during stressful times can help reduce nursing burnout and compassion fatigue.

For those nurses who are considering a return to academia, professional nursing associations offer a variety of online courses and certifications that help advance the profession through continued education opportunities. Nurses interested in specialty areas can access current courses to advance their learning and to enhance their skills. The flexible schedule of online courses provides an opportunity for personal and professional growth for nurses who would not otherwise be able to attend in-person classes.

Maintaining the Quality of Patient Care: The New Seven P's of Nursing

In the dynamic world of health, nursing is identified as an essential element of quality care (Harrison, 2024). Penny Harrison, England's chief nursing officer, has developed a strategic vision framework. In describing the "7 P's of nursing," Harrison integrates the collective, expressed aspiration of nurses worldwide to continually improve patient outcomes, while generating an inspired and invested nursing workforce. These seven components are defined below:

- **Purpose**. This element stresses the value of understanding the central mission of nursing: to provide compassionate and effective patient care. Nurses are provided guidance and support in learning to align their personal purpose with the broader goals of patient care and health outcomes.
- **Professionalism**. In promoting continuous education, ethical practices, and accountability among nurses, the intent here is to maintain the highest standards of professional conduct among nurses. This initiative strives to ensure that nurses are getting the professional credit and recognition they deserve.
- **Personalization**. In individualizing the delivery of care, nurses consider those cultural, emotional, and psychological factors that can build stronger bonds between nurses and patients, fostering better health outcomes.
- **Proactivity**. Nurses are encouraged to take charge of their own personal and professional challenges. Periodic self-assessment, attendance at continuing education classes, and adopting an attitude of openness to the perspectives of others can refresh and enhance skill sets.
- **Partnership**. Collaboration among health care providers builds stronger bonds among professionals, fosters current knowledge, and reinforces vested interests in improving patient outcomes. Partnerships may include coworkers, supervisors, stakeholders, and community members.
- **Prevention**. Identifying and managing patient health risks early on in the nurse patient relationship saves valuable time and enhances everyone's safety. The effective nurse

leader uses observational and critical thinking skills to intervene and achieve positive patient outcomes.

- **Productivity.** Improving workflow is a team effort. Nurses organize on their feet. They make effective use of the skills and resources of the people around them. Assisted with current technology, recognizing their team members' talents, and tapping into the influence and expertise of administration, nurses embrace efficiency, all while maintaining high-quality care. Productivity ensures that nursing resources are utilized to their best potential for the common goal of achieving quality patient outcomes.

Expanding the Nursing Pipeline

Resolving the current nursing shortage poses a complex challenge, but there is hope for the future. Collaborative input and efforts, from all levels and disciplines in health care organizations, to address root causes, together with innovative recruitment and retention strategies, can result in building a sustainable pipeline of skilled nurses. From expanding education capacity and offering flexible scheduling, to fostering a positive workplace culture and leveraging technology, these efforts will ensure that the nursing profession remains resilient and capable of meeting future health care demands.

Investing in the nursing workforce is critical to safeguarding the health and well-being of communities. Policymakers and health care organizations must take immediate action by prioritizing funding, supporting education initiatives, and implementing workplace reforms to build and maintain a healthy and sustainable nursing pipeline. Confronting the nursing shortage requires schools and health care providers to recruit new nurses and support working conditions that reduce turnover. Organizations such as federal and state governments, career and health advocacy organizations, have developed programs to attract and retain nurses. One example is the Nursing Education Loan Repayment Program (https://bhw.hrsa.gov/funding/apply-loan-repayment/nurse-corps), which repays up to 85% of educational loans for nurses who work in qualifying facilities in areas with critical nursing shortages.

Used to attract and inspire young people to consider a future in nursing, the "career pipeline" partners high schools with universities and colleges in venues such as nursing career fairs, shadowing programs, and scholarships. These initiatives introduce students to the health care field and the wide array of areas in the discipline to explore. Beyond financial incentives, perks such as tuition reimbursement, student loan forgiveness, and flexible scheduling can help reduce the fear often associated with applying to college.

Social media offers an efficient and effective online recruitment strategy to introduce potential nursing students to a particular program. Easily accessed on the college/university web site, this resource efficiently summarizes information, showcasing a nursing program's curriculum, clinical setting locations, program success rates (National Council Licensure Examination (NCLEX) scores) career outcomes, and student testimonials, as well as emphasizing professional development opportunities, extracurricular activities, and support networks available to students.

Professional development opportunities are critical for retaining nurses. Health care facilities can establish mentorship programs, leadership training, and continuing education opportunities to help nurses advance in their careers. Clear pathways for growth, such as transitioning from bedside nursing to management or specialty roles, can increase job satisfaction, retention, and advancement in the profession.

Transition to Practice

Several factors have been listed as reasons for the nursing shortage, including burnout, high patient-to-nurse ratios, workplace violence, work-life balance, lack of education and support, and stress related to transition into practice. With healthcare becoming more complex, and new nurses lacking confidence to practice, organizations are finding an increasing need for transition to practice (TTP) programs (Lee, 2024).

A formal program for new graduate registered nurses (NGRNs), TTP utilizes active learning to support progression from pre-licensure nursing education into licensed practice. More hospitals are recognizing the importance of TTP programs on clinical skill development, practice readiness, and socialization of their NGRNs. Rush et al. (2019) found that providing NGRNs with evidence-based, standardized, TTP programs decreased turnover and increased retention. TTP programs that incorporate targeted classroom education, computer-based learning, clinical precepted time, and mentoring offer NGRNs optimal learning experiences.

Reflective Questions

After reading this and other chapters in the book:

1. Are you feeling closer to a career decision?
2. What questions remain unanswered?
3. What additional information is needed?
4. What initially generated your interest in nursing?
5. What personal experiences have inspired you to consider a career in nursing?
6. What aspects of nursing are most appealing to you?
7. Are you prepared to be a lifelong learner?
8. What support systems do you feel foster success for a nursing student?
9. Are there any aspects of nursing that you find particularly challenging?

Scenario

The Nursing Interview

When seeking admission to nursing school, applicants often have the opportunity to meet with program representatives. Interviewers are interested in determining applicants' passion for nursing, their interpersonal skills, and their career goals. Preparing in advance your responses to potential interview questions posed can calm nerves and contribute to making an effective first impression. These questions may include the following:

1. Why do you want to become a nurse?
2. What made you choose this school in your search of nursing programs?
3. What do you consider the most important characteristic for a nurse to possess?
4. What makes you a good candidate for the nursing program?
5. Were you ever a patient? Did this experience affect your decision to become a nurse?

Health Care Experience

During an interview, a program representative may ask you about your experience in the health care field. Some of the most common questions include:

1. Do you have any certifications in healthcare (nurse's aide, home health aide)?
2. Do you have job experience in caring for people?
3. Do any family members work in healthcare? Did this inspire you to pursue nursing?
4. Describe a stressful event at work or at school, and how you responded to the pressure.

Questions the Applicant Should Ask

1. How does this program prepare students for the NCLEX?
2. What are the program's NCLEX scores for the past 5 years?
3. What are the program's retention and graduation rates?
4. Which professional accreditation agency approves this program? When was the last accreditation visit held, and what was the outcome?
5. How do you support students who are struggling (tutoring; health services)?
6. What is a typical class size? What is the instructor-to-student clinical ratio?
7. Which clinical agencies are used for student placement? Do I need my own transportation to clinical agencies?
8. How is technology used (simulation and other learning laboratories)?

The nursing school interview should showcase your communication skills, professionalism, and enthusiasm. Explain why you are excited about the field and how you see yourself contributing to nursing. Provide concrete examples from academic life, work experience, volunteering, or personal situations. In relating these experiences, emphasize essential professional skills, such as collaboration, caring, ethics, self-control under pressure, organization, and critical thinking. Come prepared with a list of questions and listen carefully to the answers provided. Remember to be your authentic self, however. The nursing interview gives you a chance to confirm that a particular program aligns with your own goals and values. Investing in nursing school shapes the trajectory of your career and your life.

Food for Thought

Removing the Elephant in the Room

"Nurses eat their young" (Gillespie et al., 2017). It is high time to retire this painful and archaic statement and rite of passage. A worn-out, harmful meme, the phrase relates to an unspoken hazing ritual of blatant lateral violence, perpetrated on students, graduates, and nurses transitioning to a new role in the discipline. It is every nurse's professional responsibility to create a welcoming, positive, and supportive environment.

Assertiveness training was not a major component of many entry-level nursing education programs. We certainly could have benefited from some form of cautionary notification (Echevarria, 2013). Replying to rude, inappropriate comments with snappy comebacks was not part of the novice nurse's repertoire. With anxiety, diminished confidence, and fear of making mistakes, bullied victims became defeated and traumatized. Many left their first positions out of nursing school, often without giving a valid reason for their exit.

Nurses became frustrated by this toxic environment and decided enough was enough. They found their voices and called out this mistreatment of "our young." Acting on the adage "if you are not part of the solution, you must be part of the problem," courageous change agents created grass roots efforts in contributing to make a difference rather than taking on the armchair spectator/critic role.

As advocates and protectors, nurses educated and supported others to fight back, to report bullying and other abusive behaviors. They shared the stories, used them in case studies and simulations, posed by the question "what would you do?" (Clark, 2017). Inservice education sessions described strategies, including promoting open communication, assertive responses, developing clear anti-bullying policies, and fostering a culture of teamwork and mentorship within health care organizations.

The research of Cynthia Clark (2023) represents ground-breaking work on fostering civility and healthy work environments. In her work, Clark identifies best practices to prevent, measure and address academic and workplace incivility. Clark proposes integrating civility, professionalism, and ethical practice concepts early on in nursing curricula in order to expose students to the benefits of healthy learning and working environments. Faculty's emphasis of these concepts during student orientation, reiterating their value during that first semester of class, incorporating into the curricula active learning strategies throughout the program, emphasizes the importance of maintaining this consistent behavior practice.

The future of nursing will require an informed, assertive, and diversified workforce, prepared to provide care, to promote positive communication among nurses, patients, families, and communities, and to address continuing health care disparities. Nurses working in the trenches can share evidence with management to inspire leaders' support of this imperative for change (Clark, 2023).

A major goal of the Committee on the Future of Nursing 2020–2030 lies in achieving health equity. In doing so, nurses contribute to initiating and maintaining equitable patient care in health care systems. To achieve health equity, the committee see the nursing profession's role as aligning public health, healthcare, social services, and public policies to eliminate health disparities and achieve health equity (National Academies of Science Engineering and Medicine, 2021).

The nation will never fully prosper until all populations are able to "live the healthiest possible life." This can be accomplished by engaging the education, experience, and expertise of all nurses in all levels and settings of the discipline to develop healthy communities for all populations. Nurses are "bridge builders" (National Academies of Science Engineering and Medicine, 2021). With ongoing collaborative support and encouragement from the organizations that educate and employ them, nurses will continue to unite people, communities, and organizations through their diligent efforts to advance health and well-being (National Academies of Science Engineering and Medicine, 2021).

References

Clark, C. M. (2017). An evidence-based approach to integrate civility, professionalism, and ethical practice into nursing curricula. *Nurse Educator*, *42*(3), 120–126. https://doi.org/10.1097/NNE.0000000000000331

Clark, C. M. (2023). Implementing trauma-informed teaching & learning principles in nursing education. *Journal of Nursing Education*, *62*(3), 133–138. doi.org/10.3928/01484834-20230109-02

Clark, C. M., Kardong-Edgren, S., & Willhaus, J. (2023). Pilot study using cognitive rehearsal, simulation, and biomarker data to address workplace incivility. *Journal of Continuing Education in Nursing*, *54*(2), 79–88. https://doi.org/10.3928/00220124-20230113-07

Echevarria, I. M. (2013). Change your appetite: Stop "eating the young" and start mentoring. *Nursing in Critical Care, 8*(3), 20–24. http://dx.doi.org/10.1097/01.CCN.0000429384.33344.2a

Gillespie, G. L., Grubb, P. L., Brown, K., Boesch, M. C., & Ulrich, D. (2017). Nurses eat their young: A novel bullying educational program for student nurses. *Journal of Nursing Education and Practice*, *7*(7), 11–21. https://doi.org/10.5430/jnep.v7n7P11

Harrison, P. (2024). England's chief nursing officer 7Ps: A new nursing framework *Gastrointestinal Nursing, 22*(2). https://doi.org/10.12968/gasn.2024.22.2.124

Lee, M. (2024). Improving new graduate nurse retention with a transition to emergency nursing practice program. *Journal of Emergency Nursing, 50*(2), 178–186. https://doi.org/10.1371/journal.pone.0230793

National Academies of Science Engineering and Medicine. (2021). *The future of nursing 2020–2030: Charting a path to achieve health equity*.The National Academies Press.https://doi/org/10.17226/2598
Rush, K., Janke, R., Duchscher, J., Phillips, R., & Kaur, S. (2019). Best practices of formal new graduate transition programs: An integrative review. *International Journal Nursing Studies. 94*,139–158. https://doi.org/10.1016/j.ijnurstu.2019. 02.010

EPILOGUE

In Memory of James Louis Duphily

I have been inspired by many events in life to write this book. But the recent loss of my son compelled me to actually put words on paper. As a mother and a nurse, I always held a subconscious obsession that my children might predecease me. When the unthinkable happened, when my son James passed away at the age of 35, I did not believe our family would survive. But here we are, a few months later, finding our way. James has passed away, but we all still feel his presence daily.

About James

James was surrounded by a large and loving extended family. He was a very smart, funny, and quick-witted guy who made friends easily. He loved camping, hiking, the ocean, scary movies, all of the holidays, and continually pranking his nieces and nephews. James would tell new friends that he was someone who came from a small rural town in Massachusetts, raised by a nurse and mechanical engineer, who instilled the values of family, hard work, self-reliance, and education into their three sons and daughter. He grew up working on cars and tractors, cutting and stacking wood, sharing cooking duties and home repair projects, and doing his own laundry(!).

As an attorney, James spent much of his legal career representing the vulnerable in society. His personal struggles fostered his ability to empathize deeply with segments of the population who deal with addiction and lack of access to effective legal resources. James was an active member of his community with volunteer work, enabling him to see firsthand these challenges in the justice system. At the time of his death, James was an attorney for a Boston law firm.

Each time I sit down to write, James is by my side, encouraging me. With an undergraduate degree in English and as an attorney, James had a gift for words. I reviewed his college and law school papers; he critiqued my doctoral work. I often wonder if I am convincing myself that writing about a loss of this magnitude will accelerate this grief journey. We nurses are impatient. We are used to multitasking, making repairs and decisions quickly, and moving on to the next challenge. But with grief, is there really a "time to move on"? I have asked this question over and over to those friends, family and colleagues who have lost loved ones. Their presence and their stories inspire and comfort. They always seem to find the right words.

I have studied grief for years. I saw it often in bedside nursing. I taught grief concepts to nursing students. Elizabeth Kübler-Ross was my guide. I now look at grief in a new way, but it is difficult to articulate, to provide a concrete description of this experience. I am asked often, "How are you feeling?" My best response is that, for me, feelings of grief come in "waves." That first trip to the grocery store after James's death was my introduction to this experience. As I passed his favorite foods, my heart beat out of my chest as if someone had jumped out at me from behind the cereal aisle.

I love hearing the funny stories about James. When followed by open arms and a hug from the storyteller, though, I became a soaking wet sponge being wrung out. Tears flowed like a monsoon, which would make some people regret that they made me cry. Others encouraged me to cry, that it would help, and it did, and still does. But for that first month, I would shop early in the morning or late at night. It has lessened somewhat, and I am venturing out more, with scripted replies as to how we all are faring.

I now recognize that my years of working in nursing and experiencing other people's grief may have compartmentalized my feelings to protect thinking about the inevitable loss of those I love. I never really understood or reflected on what loss truly means. Does that make me lucky? In our family, we remained virtually unscathed by sudden death. My grandparents and parents lived long and healthy lives. Professionally, I worked in pediatrics, maternity, med surg, and community health nursing, experiencing the life cycle journey on a pretty regular basis. You would think I would have a handle on working through grief. But losing my son was a completely different experience. I cannot predict how I will feel from one day to the next.

I have always been told how "strong" I am. I guess to most observers I weathered personal and professional storms rather easily. My husband, too, was always a veritable Rock of Gibraltar during most of life's curves. The loss of James brought us to our knees. Enter the "cavalry," my three adult children and five grandchildren (ages 8–16 years), my two daughters-in-law and my son-in-law, my siblings, my friends, and our community, to help. They arrived on the spot, loaded with food and supplies, tears and hugs, and silently went to work. My kids made brave and heartfelt speeches at the cemetery, organized the obligatory appointments, picked out the headstone, found a musician and a caterer. My daughters-in-law and son-in-law never stopped helping and caring, quietly blending in behind the scenes, picking up the load, in full protective mode. My five grandchildren stood by us at the cemetery, stoic and graceful, holding our hands. Siblings and their families welcomed visitors, washed dishes, served food and drinks, and stayed behind to pick up the pieces, literally and figuratively.

I am in complete awe of my children's courage, spirit, and unconditional love in the face of the devastating loss of their brother. They took charge when their parents could not. When did they become adults? Friends loaned us a huge tent, tables and chairs for our backyard, gifted us a housecleaner and local police to do "detail" and direct traffic to and from our home. The house overflowed with paper products, food, and drinks. Every day. People saved us.

From reading about the five stages of loss (Kübler-Ross, *On Death and Dying*) I have intellectualized grief over the years. I do recall Kübler-Ross clarifying for the reader that we move back and forth between stages in the process of grief and that grieving takes many paths foreach person. I see this clearly now. I take comfort in writing and have pictures of happy memories of the family everywhere in the house. For my husband, pictures make him sad. He finds the music he shared with James really helps his grief as he copes. When I hear these same songs, I need to leave the room.

Clothing is another area of solace for all of us, it seems. James's brothers, nieces, and nephews now share his prized and hoarded collection of "antique sneakers." James's high school friends chose some of his favorite clothes as keepsakes. My husband wears James's clothes. I value his soccer uniforms from high school and college. We both visit James'sgrave daily—it is just up the street from our home, high on a hill, surrounded by nature and the birch trees he loved. We both think of him every day. That is a good thing, I feel. We will always remember our son.

For those who encounter the person who has lost a loved one, it is okay to say, "I don't know what to say." "What can I do?" You will get an answer, guaranteed! Share your stories about the loved one who has passed and continue the dialogue the next time you meet. Saying nothing/avoiding those who have lost a loved one is hurtful. Don't be afraid to mention the name of the individual who has died when you meet that person's family members. Have gratitude for the people surrounding you and what they mean in your life—and tell them that. You can never take enough photos. Most of all, be kind.

In her speech at the Celebration of Life, friend and colleague Ashley remembers James thorough the writings of Theodore Roosevelt (1910) about "striving valiantly and daring greatly":

> *It is not the critic who counts ... not the man who points out how the strong man stumbles or where the doer of deeds could have done better.*
> *The credit belongs to the man who is actually in the arena,*
> *whose face is marred by dust and sweat and blood, who strives valiantly,*
> *who errs and comes up short again and again,*
> *because there is no effort without error or shortcoming,*
> *but who knows the great enthusiasms, the great devotions,*
> *who spends himself in a worthy cause;*
> *who, at the best, knows, in the end, the triumph of high achievement,*
> *who, at the worst, if he fails, at least he fails while daring greatly,*
> *so his place shall never be with those cold and timid souls who knew neither victory nor defeat.*

Six months after the death of our son, we attended the wedding of our youngest child. James was to be his brother's best man. Both the bride and groom felt that his role should not be replaced. A chair was placed at the ceremony in his honor. Speakers at the wedding recalled poignant (and funny) memories of a life lived to the fullest, acknowledging our son in the most appropriate and respectful manner. In no way did it dampen this beautiful celebration. Family and friends shared a common belief that James was with us at the event. His light lives on, strengthened by the continued love, support, and recognition of his time with us.

INDEX

0-9

7 P's of nursing, 132

A

Abdellah, Faye, 55
active learning, 116
    technology-based learning, 117
active listening, 30
ADPIE, 7
adverse events, 95
ART model, 96
    acknowledgment, 96
    recognition, 97
    turning, 97
artificial intelligence (AI), 11

B

bedside shift reporting (BSR), 96
behavioral systems model, 45
    homeostasis, 45
Benner, Patricia, 22, 82
blame-free environment, 93
bullying, 92
burnout, 38, 67, 92, 132
    symptoms, 92

C

caring, 29
Caritas Processes, 31
change, 21
    resistance, 21
change theory, 23
    change, 24
    change shock, 24
    driving forces, 23
    equilibrium, 24
    refreezing, 24
    restraining forces, 23
    unfreezing, 24
    unfreezing-change-refreeze model, 24
chief nursing officer (CNO), 78
civility, 53, 91
    operating room teamwork, 53
clinical practice guideline (CPGs), 128
Cochrane, Archibald, 7
comfort theory, 70
compassion fatigue, 38, 92
    risk factors, 92
continuing education, 131
    continuing education units (CEUs), 10
Core Competencies of Nurse Educators (NLN), 84
COVID-19 pandemic, 67, 77
critical incidents, 21
    theory-practice links, 21
critical thinking, 8
cultural assessment, 104
cultural awareness, 43, 103
    biases, 43
    cultural self-awareness, 106
cultural competence, 43, 105
    stereotyping, 43
cultural difference, 103
cultural dissonance, 103
    communication barriers, 103
cultural humility, 43
    self-reflection, 43
cultural knowledge, 106
cultural literacy, 104
    lifelong process, 105
cultural sensitivity, 43, 45
cultural stigma, 44
culturally congruent care, 46
culturally responsive care, 44
culture of safety, 91

D

duty to provide care
    personal risk, 53

E

electronic health records (EHR), 64, 118
electronic medical records (EMR), 118
empathy, 29
end-of-life care, 39, 70
environmental theory of nursing, 3
    patient care, 54
equitable care, 45
evidence-based practice (EBP), 8, 37, 127

F

five stages of grief theory, 39
food insecurity, 108
    food desert, 108
functional health patterns, 6

G

Gordon, Marjory, 6
Gottlieb, Laurie, 54

H

Haiti, 50
head, heart, and hands, 4
    affective, 4
    cognitive, 4
    psychomotor, 5
health-seeking behavior, 46
Healthy People 2030, 109
HIV/AIDS, 47
holism, 110
holistic approach, 29, 33
holistic nursing care, 110
    staffing shortages, 110
humor, 25
    nursing practice, 26
    patient care, 26
    therapeutic uses, 26

I

I-PASS, 96
identification phase, 68
incivility, 53, 91
informatics, 115, 118
    informatics literacy, 115
    information systems, 115
information literacy, 117
interpersonal process, 68
interpersonal relation theory, 30
interpreter services, 52
interprofessional collaboration, 93
intuition, 59, 61
    decision-making, 59
    emotional intelligence, 61
    information prioritization, 61
    pattern recognition, 61
    prior experience, 61
    research, 61

J

Johnson, Dorothy, 45
just culture, 95

K

Kangaroo Mother Care, 48
King, Imogene, 40
Kolcaba, Katherine, 70
Kotter's (1996) Eight Step Change Model, 116
    clear vision, 116
    sense of urgency, 116
    short-term wins, 116
Kurt Lewin's change theory, 125
    driving forces, 125
    equilibrium, 125
    restraining forces, 125
Kübler-Ross, Elisabeth, 39

L

Leininger, Madeleine, 104
    culture care theory, 46
Lewin, Kurt, 23
lifelong learning, 59, 131
    continuing professional development (CPD), 59
    principles, 65

M

Mandela, Nelson, 48
medical mission, 50
mentoring, 81
    collegial mentoring model, 81
Mothers Programmes, 48

N

Neuman, Betty
    environmental stressors, 60
    systems model, 60
Nightingale, Florence, 3
    healing process, 54
Notes on Hospitals (Nightingale), 4
Notes on Nursing (Nightingale), 3
novice to expert, 82
novice to expert theory, 22
    competent, 22
    novice, 22
nurse-patient relationship, 30
nursing education, 4
nursing informatics specialist (NIS), 118
    data analytics, 118
    informatics literacy, 119
    patient safety and privacy, 119
nursing pipeline, 133
nursing process, 5, 62
    assessment, 5
    diagnosis, 5
    evaluation, 6
    implementation, 6
    outcomes/planning, 6
nursing shortage, 77, 133
    nursing education faculty shortage, 85
nursing theory, 37, 68

P

palliative care, 70
passing the torch, 10
patient advocacy, 45
patient fall, 126
patient-centered care, 12, 37, 45, 77, 123
peaceful death, 70
Peplau, Hildegard, 30, 68
person-centered care, 94
Picker, Harvey, 12
    Picker Survey, 12
PICOT, 8
Plan-Do-Study-Act (PDSA) cycle, 124
professional development, 133

Q

quality improvement (QI), 123, 126
    quality improvement (QI) model, 123

R

resilience, 67, 97
    activation, 67
    decompression, 67
    leadership strategies, 67
Robben Island, 48
Rogers, Martha, 46
Root Cause Analysis (RCA), 124
Roy, Callista
    adaptation model, 63
    physiologic-physical mode, 64
    role function, 64

S

SBAR, 96
science of unitary human beings, 46
    holistic assessment, 46
self-care, 31, 68
shared decision-making, 40
social determinants of health (SDOH), 107
    health inequities, 108
South Africa, 47
strengths-based nursing care
    family support, 54
Strengths-Based Nursing Care: Health and Healing for Person and Family (Gottlieb), 54
Supplemental Nutrition Assistance Program (SNAP), 108
Swanson, Kristen
    caring model, 62
    therapeutic relationships, 62

T

telehealth, 11, 117
    nursing quality, 117
    remote monitoring, 117
the four C's of culture model, 105
theory of goal attainment, 40
theory of human caring, 31, 37
theory of transpersonal caring, 23
    carative factors, 23
transcultural nursing concept, 104
transition to practice, 79, 134
twenty-one nursing problems
    patient-centered approach, 55

V

vulnerable populations, 70

W

Watson, Jean, 23, 29, 31, 62
    caring theory, 62
    patient-centered care, 62
wearable devices, 118
workplace violence, 53, 91
    home care, 53
    prevalence, 92